T0144867

BASIC HEALTH PUBLICATIONS USER'S GUIDE

TO HEALTHY DIGESTION

Learn How You Can Put an End to Heartburn, Indigestion, Constipation, and Other Digestive Problems.

VICTORIA DOLBY TOEWS, M.P.H.

JACK CHALLEM Series Editor

The information contained in this book is based upon the research and personal and professional experiences of the author. It is not intended as a substitute for consulting with your physician or other healthcare provider. Any attempt to diagnose and treat an illness should be done under the direction of a healthcare professional.

The publisher does not advocate the use of any particular healthcare protocol but believes the information in this book should be available to the public. The publisher and author are not responsible for any adverse effects or consequences resulting from the use of the suggestions, preparations, or procedures discussed in this book. Should the reader have any questions concerning the appropriateness of any procedures or preparations mentioned, the author and the publisher strongly suggest consulting a professional healthcare advisor.

Series Editor: Jack Challem
Editor: Carol Rosenberg
Typesetter: Gary A. Rosenberg
Series Cover Designer: Mike Stromberg

Basic Health Publications User's Guides are published by Basic Health Publications, Inc.

ISBN: 978-1-59120-085-7 (Pbk.)
ISBN: 978-1-68162-857-8 (Hardcover)

CONTENTS

INTRODUCTION

The enjoyment of a good meal is one of life's pleasures. When the gut works right, as with most organs, we don't notice it. Unfortunately, trouble can start brewing as soon as a mouthful of your favorite dish is swallowed. Faulty digestion causes a lot of unnecessary discomfort due to heartburn, bloating, gas, and sour stomach. Digestion problems also contribute to many gastrointestinal and related health problems, such as irritable bowel syndrome, peptic ulcer, and Crohn's disease.

Everything we eat must be broken down, absorbed, assimilated, and finally eliminated. Problems at any of these steps bring the whole digestive process to a grinding halt, leaving the body vulnerable to nutritional deficiencies, toxic buildup, and overall poor health.

Digestion-related illnesses exert a considerable toll on comfort, health, quality of life, and your pocketbook. If you feel like food (and your body's processing of it) has become your enemy, this book is for you.

You'll learn how to prevent and manage indigestion in Chapter 1, and Chapter 2 will cover the exceedingly common problems of constipation, diarrhea, and irritable bowel syndrome. Move along to Chapter 3 to learn about food allergies, lactose intolerance, celiac disease, and leaky gut syndrome, and then to Chapter 4 to relieve your nausea and vomiting. Chapters 5, 6, 7, and 8 will review natural treatments for gallstones, liver health, hiatal hernia, cancer-risk reduction, ulcers, gastritis, and inflammatory bowel disease (Crohn's disease and ulcerative colitis). Finally, you'll want to turn to Chapter 9 if you're concerned about diverticulitis, hemorrhoids, or excessive intestinal gas.

Located at the end of the book are two helpful appendices. Appendix A is a handy chart detailing all of the dietary supplements and herbs that are useful for digestive complaints. The amount to take for each supplement or herb, as well as potential side effects, are listed. In case your high-school biology is a little rusty, Appendix B provides a refresher of how the digestive process works.

Certainly, there is much to gain from reading this book cover to cover, but if you are currently suffering from a particular problem and want to get right to it, the following index will show you which chapter to turn to for your specific health complaint:

Health Complaint	Chapter
Cancer of digestive tract	6
Celiac disease	3
Colon therapy	9
Constipation	2
Crohn's disease	8
Diarrhea	2
Diverticulitis	9
Enema	9
Food allergies	3
Food poisoning	4
Gallstones	5
Gas	9
Gastritis	7

CHAPTER 1

WAS IT SOMETHING
I ATE?

Every once in a while about half of us Americans suffer from indigestion—an umbrella term to describe symptoms such as heartburn, upset stomach, bloating, gas, and slow digestion—and 25 million Americans face indigestion as a daily part of life. It doesn't have to be this way, since there are many natural remedies for this common condition.

Causes of Indigestion

There is often no specific culprit that can be identified as a cause of indigestion. Other times, with a bit of sleuthing, you can determine the cause of your dyspepsia and take steps to remedy the underlying condition. All too often, indigestion is a condition of "too much," such as eating too much, eating too quickly, or eating while under too much stress.

Dyspepsia *Another name for indigestion.*

Obesity and pregnancy can be instigators of heartburn, since extra weight can push the stomach contents back into the esophagus. Hiatal hernias, discussed in Chapter 5, are another cause of indigestion. Medications that irritate the stomach lining (such as aspirin) can also be an underlying trigger of indigestion.

In some cases, indigestion is experienced on a persistent basis but is not related to poor diet choices or underlying diseases. This type of indigestion might be caused by a problem with the muscular squeezing action of the stomach. In such cases, a doctor might prescribe a medication to alter stomach motility (movement).

In itself, indigestion is merely a cause of discomfort but is not generally harmful to your health. However, indigestion can be a symptom of a serious disease such as peptic ulcer, gastritis, or gallbladder disease. If you suffer from chronic indigestion, it's a good idea to consult a physician to rule out the possibility that it is a sign of a more serious condition.

Indigestion can be a sign of or mimic of other serious diseases. Please consult a doctor if your indigestion is accompanied by any of the following symptoms:

- vomiting, weight loss, or loss of appetite

- black tarry stools or blood in vomit

- severe pain in the upper right abdomen

- discomfort unrelated to eating

- shortness of breath, sweating, or pain radiating to the jaw, neck, or arm

Prevention Is the Best Treatment

Avoiding the foods or situations that seem to trigger a bout of indigestion is often the best and simplest way to treat this problem. An indigestion prevention plan should be based on a wholesome, low-fat diet. Fatty foods can lead to indigestion, since they take longer to digest and result in a full, bloated feeling and even pain. Overeating is another red flag; smaller meals at regular intervals are a better choice. If indigestion is a result of a food allergy or intolerance (see Chapter 3), then avoiding the problem food can be an easy fix.

Foods and beverages (including coffee, tea, colas, and tomato-based foods) that crank up acid in the stomach should be avoided or at least minimized if they are a problem for your stomach. Alcohol and tobacco are other promoters of sour stomach. Smokers can help relieve their indigestion by stopping smoking (quitting is, of course, good for overall health) or at least not smoking right before eating.

When and how meals are eaten can be another tie to indigestion. Exercising with a full stomach is a sure way, for many people, to bring on an upset stomach. The digestive system requires a tremendous amount of blood to process food, and putting muscles to work diverts this needed blood. Scheduling exercise before a meal or waiting for an hour after eating helps keep digestion moving properly.

On the other hand, you don't want to completely shut your body down after a meal. Lying down or even slouching after a meal can bring on a bout of heartburn, since these positions increase stomach pressure. A good rule of thumb is to wait two hours after eating before going to bed. In addition, raising the head of the bed by 3 to 6 inches can help by using the force of gravity to keep the stomach in place and prevent a reflux of stomach acids.

Constipation can worsen heartburn symptoms in someone with a hiatal hernia, since straining distends the abdomen and further widens the hernia. Constipation treatment, discussed in Chapter 2, can be tried.

Heartburn and GERD

Heartburn, the most common symptom of indigestion, is a burning feeling in the chest that occurs because stomach acid and other stomach contents have flowed backward into the esophagus. This movement of stomach acid, known as reflux, irritates the esophagus because, unlike the stomach, the esophagus does not have a protective lining of mucus-producing tissue.

Gastroesophageal reflux disease, otherwise known as GERD or acid reflux, is diagnosed when heartburn is frequent or severe enough to be more than an occasional nuisance and interferes with one's quality of life or even damages the esophagus. GERD generally occurs because the sphincter between the esophagus and the stomach is not functioning properly. Along with heartburn, some people with GERD experience regurgitation of stomach acid into the mouth, difficulty swallowing, and chest pain. GERD can even cause asthma, coughing, vocal cord inflammation with hoarseness, and sore throat. GERD most commonly occurs in people over the age of forty.

Enzymes Promote Digestion

The three types of macronutrients in food—proteins, carbohydrates, and fats—each have a corresponding class of digestive enzymes that digest them. Proteolytic enzymes (or proteases) are used for digesting protein, lipases digest fat, and amylases are needed during the digestion of carbohydrates. The pancreas produces these enzymes, which is why they are collectively known as pancreatic enzymes. Inadequate production of pancreatic enzymes, which is increasingly common as the years add up, can lead to symptoms of indigestion.

Macronutrients
Food constituents that supply calories: proteins, carbohydrates, and fats.

There are tests to determine the quantity and quality of the body's production of digestive enzymes, but these tests are difficult and expensive. A simpler test is to add supplemental digestive enzymes to a meal and judge if digestion is improved. If so, continued use of digestive enzymes could go a long way in promoting good digestion. In one recent study, feelings of gas, bloating, and fullness after eating a high-fat meal were eased significantly when a time-release form of pancreatic enzymes were taken.

But knowing how much to take of the various digestive enzymes can be tricky. The government has helped by establishing a standard for the pancreatic enzymes (just as with herbal extracts), to which enzyme supplements are compared. If a supplement contains 9X pancreatic enzymes, it would provide nine times the amount of each of the enzymes (amylase, lipase, and proteolytic enzymes) in the standard.

Standardized Herbal Extracts
Herbs processed to contain consistent levels of key active substances.

As a general guideline, if a 9X enzyme supplement is used, 1.5 grams of the supplement taken with each meal should be adequate to aid in food digestion in individuals with pancreatic insufficiency. Greater amounts of a lower potency product will be needed to achieve the same effect.

Bitter Herbs for Better Digestion

While most people consume plenty of salty, sweet, and sour foods, bitter foods are eaten few and far between. Bitter herbs encourage salivation and production of stomach acid and digestive enzymes—in other words, they get your juices flowing. Because stomach acid increases with their use, bitter herbs are recommended for indigestion that is not accompanied by heartburn.

There are many herbs with bitter properties, but gentian is one of the most often used for this purpose. Others include artichoke, greater cel -

andine, dandelion, bitter orange, centaury, and blessed thistle. Bitters are particularly valuable for people who eat a lot of fatty, hard-to-digest foods.

Artichokes, in addition to being a tasty vegetable, are a mild bitter. Artichoke extract (containing the active constituent cynarin) has been demonstrated in several studies to ease symptoms of indigestion.

Additional Herbs for Indigestion

Chamomile should be one of the first herb choices when heartburn strikes. Chamomile soothes the irritation of the digestive tract and encourages normal digestion. It is most commonly used in a tea form for this purpose.

Over the centuries, herbalists have identified dozens of herbs with stomach-friendly properties. Of them, many have been scrutinized by modern medicine and confirmed to be effective to allay indigestion. For example, double-blind research has found a combination of peppermint oil (36–90 mg) and caraway oil (20–50 mg) in enteric-coated capsules to be effective for easing indigestion. Ginger is best known for making car and air travel more tolerable for those who are susceptible to motion sickness, but it has also been shown to aid digestion.

Licorice protects the mucous membranes that line the digestive tract against the damaging effects of stomach acid. This effect can be very helpful for those with heartburn. Licorice root extract in the form of deglycyrrhizinated licorice (DGL) is preferable since the glycyrrhizin component of licorice can cause high blood pressure. The glycyrrhizin is removed in the DGL form, but the ability to resolve indigestion remains in the product.

Slippery elm is another herb that acts as a barrier against stomach acid, which again is important for those with heartburn.

Why Not Just Pop an Antacid?

With millions of Americans suffering with indigestion daily, it's no surprise that peddling antacids has become quite a lucrative business. However, the use of antacids to treat heartburn and indigestion in general is questionable. Antacids suppress acid production, but in most cases, the problem is not actually whether or not there is acid, but rather that the acid is in the wrong place (such as refluxed into the esophagus). Even so, some people report that antacids do provide symptom relief (many experts would claim that they are simply experiencing the placebo effect).

If you choose to use antacids, keep in mind that their constant use can be detrimental since they interfere with the absorption of vitamins and minerals (such as folic acid and copper) and other medications. In any case, with such a cornucopia of herbs available to treat indigestion, it seems a shame not to give herbal medicine a go for indigestion relief.

Placebo Effect
When health improves because a person believes the treatment to be effective, even if a sugar pill was unknowingly the "medicine" used.

Bottom Line

- Avoid the foods or activities that trigger indigestion (for example, wolfing down a cup of black coffee as you race out the door for the day).

- Indigestion is very treatable with the use of natural remedies.

- Chamomile is an all-around stomach soother.

Other great herbs to consider include peppermint, caraway, ginger, licorice, and slippery elm.

- Pancreatic enzymes can aid the digestive process.

- Bitter herbs are great helpers for optimal digestion.

CHAPTER 2

Rushing to the Toilet or Wishing You Could Go

Any change in bowel habits can interfere with your day: either causing you to race from bathroom to bathroom or waiting around with hopes of feeling the urge to use the toilet. What is considered normal for bowel function varies widely from person to person. Normal bowel movements range from as many as three stools a day to as few as three a week.

A normal movement is one that is formed but not hard, contains no blood, and is passed without cramps or pain. If you suddenly find yourself racing to the bathroom with diarrhea, or wondering if you'll ever go again because of constipation, or perhaps alternating between the two conditions because of irritable bowel syndrome, then this chapter is for you and will help you find the right balance with your bowel.

Constipation Basics

Constipation occurs when a person has a de crease in daily bowel movements and/or passes hard, dry stool. Pain or difficulty passing the stool is common with this condition. In the vast majority of the cases, constipation is the result of poor diet choices, namely too little fiber in the diet and insufficient fluids. The sad fact is that most people would never deal with a bout of constipation if they ate right. But the way things stand with the average American diet, an estimated

10 percent of us suffer from constipation (and twice as many elderly Americans are afflicted). However, constipation can be a sign of a disease such as diverticulitis, hypothyroidism, or irritable bowel syndrome. You'll want to make sure that your doctor has ruled out such medical causes of constipation.

Fiber keeps things moving through the intestine. In addition, fiber acts as a sponge, attracting water to the stool. This doesn't necessarily mean a fiber supplement. Fiber is part of all whole grains, fruits, and vegetables. If you are suffering from constipation, the first thing you should try is to increase your intake of such foods. Wheat bran is one type of fiber that can be effective when added to the diet. Try adding a quarter cup or more of wheat bran to a breakfast cereal, or choose a high-bran cereal. But keep in mind that any increase of high-fiber foods should be gradual to help prevent bloating and gas.

Make sure you drink plenty of fluids, too—at least eight glasses a day. (Increasing fiber intake without boosting fluids can backfire and make constipation worse.) Without adequate fluids, stool becomes hard and can even develop rough edges, which can produce tiny tears in the rectum. Feel free to choose from water, juices, herbal teas, and soups, but avoid black and green teas, since they contain tannins that help bind stools. Prunes and prune juice are time-honored constipation remedies, and for good reason: they work.

Spending more time at the gym or even a simple walk around the neighborhood on occasion can help, since physical activity promotes a well-functioning bowel and stimulates the wavelike contractions of the intestines that move stool out of the body.

Even if your diet is full of fiber and fluids, you

can become constipated if you ignore the urge to have a bowel movement. Waiting allows more water to be absorbed by the large intestine, leading to harder stool that is painful to pass. Take the time to go to the bathroom as soon as you feel the urge; this helps maintain regularity.

Laxatives from the Pharmacy

There are three general categories of laxatives that a conventional doctor would recommend: bulk-forming laxatives, stimulant laxatives, and stool softeners. Bulk-forming laxatives increase the amount of bulk in the intestines, softening the stool to make it easier to pass, and initiating peristalsis. This type of laxative includes natural fibers, cellulose, and synthetic polysaccharides. Stimulant laxatives, such as disacodyl, senna, and castor oil, irritate the intestinal wall in order to stimulate peristalsis. Stool softeners, such as the medication docusate sodium, soften the stool to make it easier to pass.

Peristalsis
The rhythmic waves that move food down the esophagus, into the stomach, through the intestinal tract, and lastly out of the body as waste.

Laxatives can cause cramping and should be used with care, since they can sometimes be more effective than anticipated and result in loose bowels. While using one of these on occasion probably isn't harmful, long-term use of laxatives can weaken the colon or lead to fluid retention. Laxative abuse is most often seen in the elderly and people with eating disorders.

Herbal Laxatives

Laxatives derived from plants are the most common laxatives used worldwide. Like their pharmacy counterparts, herbal laxatives include the categories of bulk-forming laxatives and stimulant laxatives.

Psyllium, flaxseed, fenugreek, and glucomannan are all bulk-forming laxatives with a high-
fiber content that supply extra bulk to the stool.
They also contain mucilage that expands when it
comes in contact with water (which is why these
laxatives *must* be taken with plenty of water).
These herbs are fairly mild laxatives that can be
used on an ongoing basis, if desired. These bulk-
forming laxatives generally lead to a bowel
movement within twelve to twenty-four hours.

Herbal stimulants tend to be more potent than
the bulk-forming herbs. Stimulant herbs, such as
senna, cascara, and aloe, contain a natural laxative compound called anthraquinone glycosides
that stimulates contractions of the bowel muscles.
Of these herbs, cascara is the mildest. Aloe can
be very potent and should be used cautiously.
These stimulant laxative herbs should be a last
resort, only after you've tried dietary changes and
bulk-forming herbs. These herbs can also cause
dependency (that is, your bowels won't move
without them), so should be used only for short
periods of time to prevent dependency.

A combination of a bulk-forming herb and a
stimulant can also be effective. Taking senna and
psyllium together (20 percent senna and 80 percent psyllium) has been effective for some cases
of chronic constipation.

Chlorophyll is not a laxative, per se, but there
have been reports that this herbal supplement is
helpful for a wide variety of digestive complaints,
including chronic constipation.

Diarrhea: Treating "The Runs"

Episodes of loose watery stools that occur three
or more times in one day are generally considered to be diarrhea. Abdominal cramps, nausea,
vomiting, fever, loss of appetite, and bloody or
foul-smelling stools are often present, as well.

Many serious diseases can cause diarrhea (including infections that continue to rank as a leading killer of Third World children), but this discussion is limited to the common, run-of-the-mill diarrhea bouts that tend to resolve themselves within forty-eight hours. Diarrhea lasting longer than this will need to be treated by a physician, rather than with at-home remedies.

The most important thing to do for diarrhea is to stay hydrated. Diarrhea causes the body to lose lots of fluids, and this risk of dehydration is the most common medical consequence of ordinary diarrhea. It cannot be emphasized strongly enough: during diarrhea, drink lots of fluids, such as water, herbal tea, vegetable juice, or broth. (Avoid fruit juice, coffee, and caffeinated soda.)

The BRAT diet is also useful for an acute bout of diarrhea. BRAT stands for the mild, well-tolerated foods Bananas, Rice, Apples, and Toast. These foods provide nutrients such as fiber and potassium that help treat diarrhea.

As your diarrhea subsides, you'll want to continue to be gentle to your recovering intestines by eating a simple diet that is easily processed, such as carrot soup, dry cereal, crackers, mashed potatoes, or other foods that seem appetizing during your recovery. For the next day or two, avoid dairy products, high-protein foods, and fatty foods.

Check Your Diet for Diarrhea Triggers

Some people are sensitive to coffee, and drinking several cups daily can induce diarrhea. If you're a coffee drinker and regularly have trouble with diarrhea, it is worth a try to avoid all coffee for a few days to see if there is an improvement in your bowel habits.

A type of fruit sugar called sorbitol can trigger diarrhea in some sensitive people. Sorbitol is absorbed slowly, and during its stay in the intestine, sorbitol tends to hold on to water, and in this way leads to diarrhea. If you suspect that you could be reacting to sorbitol, you'll want to avoid it by reading labels for this ingredient and avoiding those foods, as well as fruit juice, to see if this simple change eliminates your problem.

Sorbitol
A sugar found in some fruits, such as apples and pears. Some dietetic candies contain sorbitol.

Taking too much of the dietary supplements vitamin C or magnesium can sometimes be a cause of diarrhea. The amount that is problematic varies for each individual, and other signs of illness, such as fever, does not accompany the diarrhea. More than a few grams per day of vitamin C are generally needed to initiate a problem; however, many people are not bothered by ten times this amount. For magnesium, most people do not have a problem until intake exceeds 350–500 mg per day. Keep in mind that magnesium-containing laxatives are a source of magnesium and taking too much for constipation can end up causing diarrhea.

Antibiotic-induced Diarrhea

The use of antibiotics has been a double-edged sword. Since their discovery early in the twentieth century, antibiotics have cured previously incurable diseases and saved countless lives. However, antibiotics kill the helpful bacteria along with the bad, leaving your intestinal tract devoid of its important friendly flora. The friendly flora help control the overgrowth of disease-causing organisms.

When the good bacteria, called probiotics, that usually reside in the intestine are killed off, diarrhea often results. Replenishing supplies of beneficial bacteria is important after a course of antibiotics. Active culture yogurt or supplements providing beneficial bacteria can also be taken as a preventative during antibiotic use. In fact, taking probiotic supplements to replace the beneficial bacteria can cut in half your chances of antibiotic-induced diarrhea. (See Chapter 9 for a more complete discussion of the friendly probiotic bacteria that are found in the intestines.)

Even if antibiotic use is not the reason for an episode of diarrhea, the diarrhea itself flushes out intestinal microorganisms, leaving the body vulnerable to opportunistic infections. Replacing the flushed out healthy bacteria with probiotic supplements is important in preventing new infections. Restoring the body's natural balance of probiotic bacteria will help ensure a smoothly running digestive tract.

Probiotics
Helpful bacteria that are found in the intestine, active culture yogurt, and dietary supplements.

Traveler's diarrhea, caused by harmful bacteria in drinking water or undercooked foods, is suffered by about 20 to 30 percent of tourists. Probiotic supplements have been found to prevent "Montezuma's revenge" in up to 90 percent or more of travelers.

Replacing Lost Nutrients

The outflow of digestive contents that occurs with diarrhea can lead to deficiencies of many vitamins and minerals, since food is rushed through the system so fast that the body doesn't have time to process it. Consequently, it's a good idea to take a general-purpose multivitamin/mineral supplement during and after a bout of diarrhea. In particular, you'll want to make sure that you're taking enough of the B vitamin folic acid. This vitamin helps to repair the lining of the intestine that may have been damaged during an episode of diarrhea.

Brewer's yeast supplements can quell diarrhea by fighting off infectious organisms. (Brewer's yeast is not the same as nutritional or torula yeast; when buying this product at a store, make sure you have real brewer's yeast.) *Saccharo - myces boulardii* is an organism related to brewer's yeast that is widely used in Europe to prevent diarrhea resulting from antibiotic use, as well as preventing traveler's diarrhea.

Herbal Diarrhea Remedies

Numerous herbs can be helpful in treating loose bowels. The antidiarrheal herbs generally contain one or more of three basic ingredients: tannin, pectin, or mucilage. Tannins are compounds in herbs that act as astringents. The astringency of tannins is the reason they lessen intestinal inflammation. Pectin adds bulk to stool because it is a soluble fiber. Mucilage also adds bulk, but it does it in a different way—by absorbing water and swelling in size. Mucilage also soothes the digestive tract.

Astringent
A compound that has the ability to bind up or contract tissues.

Carob is a prime example of an herb that provides tannins. Carob can be used for adult cases of diarrhea, as well as cases that occur in children or infants. Other astringent herbs include blackberry and red raspberry. The leaves of these two herbs can be used to make an astringent tea. Bilberry in the form of dried berries or juice also provides tannins, but the fresh berries should not be used because they can worsen diarrhea. Both green tea and black tea are very astringent and fit the bill for a beverage of choice during diarrhea.

Apple pulp is a great source of pectin, which explains why apples and applesauce have long been recommended in the diets of those recovering from diarrhea. Psyllium seeds add bulk to stool and can help resolve diarrhea symptoms.

Mucilage-providing herbs include marshmallow and slippery elm. These can be very soothing to the digestive tract. Fenugreek seeds are another rich source of mucilage, but they should be limited to two teaspoons at a time, otherwise they may induce abdominal distress.

Irritable Bowel Syndrome (IBS)

Irritable bowel syndrome (IBS) is characterized by crampy pain, bloating, gas, and altered bowel habits. People with IBS often alternate between constipation and diarrhea. It is not known what causes IBS, and it has proved difficult to treat with conventional medicine. For some people, IBS is just a mild annoyance, but for others, it is disabling since they cannot be far from a bathroom.

The good news, if it can be called such, is that although IBS causes a great deal of discomfort and distress, it doesn't lead to any permanent harm to the intestines, intestinal bleeding, or to a serious disease such as cancer.

Searching for a Cause of IBS

Although stress was once thought to be the cause of IBS, it is now known that emotional conflict and stress do not cause the disease. Stress does, however, worsen symptoms. Many people report more intense symptoms of IBS while under stress. Relaxation techniques or counseling help relieve IBS symptoms in some people.

The colon normally experiences contractions that move food along during the digestive process. If the colon contracts too strongly or too weakly, symptoms result. Chocolate, dairy products, sorbitol, alcohol, or caffeine are foods that many people report cause these erratic colon contractions. Avoiding dairy products or taking lactase enzyme supplements with dairy products relieves IBS symptoms for some people. You'll want to keep track of any foods that seem to be triggers for you, and try avoiding these foods to see if you feel better.

In addition, fat is a trigger for colon spasms and the more fat in a meal, the more likely that meal is to cause an episode of discomfort. Large meals, regardless of their fat content, can also cause problems. Stick to smaller portions eaten more often. A multivitamin/mineral supplement might be a good idea to provide some nutritional insurance against deficiencies that may be caused by poor digestion.

Conversely, the diet can help minimize the recurrence of IBS. Dietary fiber is helpful to many people with IBS. Including such foods as whole-grain breads and cereals, beans, fruits, and vegetables in the diet is a good idea. Slowly increase the amount of fiber in your diet; adding too much, too fast can cause gas and bloating. However, a slow increase will avoid this problem. Wheat bran as a source of fiber has been reported in some research to make people feel worse, which may indicate that wheat allergy is common in IBS.

Fiber supplements are sometimes recommended to address the constipation of IBS. Psyllium seeds have been studied in this regard and have been shown to improve symptoms of IBS.

Herbal Answers for IBS

Peppermint is a general digestive aid, and it is certainly called for in cases of IBS. Peppermint lessens the production of gas, eases intestinal cramps, and soothes irritated tissues. Several studies have reported that peppermint oil makes IBS symptoms better. Most research has used the enteric-coated capsule form of peppermint oil, which ensures that the oil is released in the intes-

tines instead of the stomach. The generally recommended amount is 0.2–0.4 ml of peppermint
oil taken three times per day, but take a bit less if
you have a burning sensation when you move
your bowels. Some dietary supplements are
available that include caraway oil in the enteric-
coated capsules. This combination has also been
successfully studied in relieving IBS symptoms.

There is some evidence that artichoke leaf
extract might be useful for dyspepsia, a condition
that shares some common symptoms as IBS. As
such, a six-week post-marketing surveillance study
of artichoke leaf extract was undertaken. A subgroup of individuals with dyspeptic symptoms
who were taking artichoke leaf extract was identified as having IBS symptoms. This subgroup
was found to have significant reductions in their
symptom severity. In fact, 96 percent of the subjects considered artichoke leaf extract to be as
good as or better than any previous IBS therapy
they had used.

Another all-around digestive-friendly herb is
chamomile. Feel free to give this gentle herb a
try for your IBS symptoms.

Women with IBS sometimes have their worst
symptoms just before and during menstruation. If
so, evening primrose oil (supplying 360–400 mg
of gamma-linolenic acid) each day has been
found to help.

Bottom Line

- For constipation, consider trying bulk-forming
  laxatives, such as psyllium, flaxseed, fenugreek,
  or glucomannan; stimulant laxatives, such as
  senna, cascara, or aloe; or chlorophyll.

- For diarrhea, some great natural remedies
  include probiotics, brewer's yeast, *Saccharomyces boulardii*, carob, blackberry, green tea,

psyllium, marshmallow, slippery elm, or fenu-greek.

- For irritable bowel syndrome, many people have found relief with peppermint oil/caraway, artichoke, chamomile, or evening primrose oil.

CHAPTER 3

WHEN FOOD
BITES BACK

For all too many people, eating is no longer the enjoyable experience it should be. Food allergies or sensitivities, as well as lactose intolerance, a reaction to gluten in grains, impaired ability to absorb nutrients, or a "leaky" gut leave many people feeling ill when they leave the dinner table. This chapter will help restore some of the enjoyment of eating.

Allergic Reactions to Food

Food allergies provoke an immune reaction when certain foods are consumed. Food sensitivities, such as lactose intolerance, do not involve the immune system, but there is an unpleasant reaction to a food, nonetheless. Most food allergies and sensitivities cause bothersome but relatively mild to moderate symptoms such as nausea, vomiting, diarrhea, constipation, indigestion, headaches, skin rashes or hives, itching, and/or shortness of breath. Fortunately, life-threatening allergic reactions called anaphylaxis are uncommon, but can occur in people who are allergic to peanuts and other nuts or shellfish.

Anaphylaxis
Severe allergic response in which the airway can narrow to the point that breathing is difficult or even impossible.

Common food allergens include wheat, soy, dairy products, eggs, corn, citrus fruits, nuts (including peanuts), tomatoes, food colorings, food preservatives, chocolate, fish, and shellfish.

An estimated 2 percent of adults and 5 to 8 percent of children are allergic to one or more foods. As these numbers show, food allergies are more common in infants and children, but often lessen as the child matures and can disappear by adulthood. Food allergies do run in families, however, and having one or both parents with an allergy greatly increases the chances that the child will have food allergies.

Table 3.1 below lists common allergenic foods and their symptoms.

TABLE 3.1. COMMON FOOD ALLERGIES AND REACTIONS	
ALLERGENIC FOOD	**COMMON SYMPTOMS (IN DESCENDING ORDER OF PREVALENCE)**
Milk and other dairy products	Diarrhea, constipation, vomiting
Eggs (especially egg whites)	Hives or other rash, swelling, upset stomach, asthma, eczema
Fish	Hives or other rash, asthma
Shellfish	Nausea, upset stomach, migraine, rash, anaphylaxis
Wheat	Diarrhea, upset stomach, migraine, eczema
Corn	Hives or other rash, difficulty breathing, diarrhea, upset stomach
Peanuts and other nuts	Upset stomach, difficulty breathing, anaphylaxis
Soy	Runny nose, diarrhea, upset stomach, hives or other rash
Citrus fruits	Hives or rash on the face, itching and tingling in the mouth
Tomatoes	Heartburn, headache
Chocolate	Hives or other rash
Food coloring/ preservatives	Headaches, asthma, hyperactivity

Tracking Down Food Allergies

Most allergic reactions show up within a few minutes or hours after eating the food. In some cases, however, the reaction may be delayed up to forty-eight hours, which can make it difficult to track down the food culprit. It can be useful to keep a food diary that notes the time and content of all foods that you eat, along with the time that any symptoms appeared. Over the course of a week or two, a pattern might emerge. Try avoiding the suspected food for at least a week, while keeping an eye on any symptoms, and then reintroduce the food to see if any symptoms reoccur.

In more complicated cases, or when multiple food allergies are suspected, it might be easier to start out with an allergy test. A nutritionist or other healthcare professional can administer a food allergy test, such as a skin prick or blood test. Afterward, a technique called elimination/provocation can be used to confirm which foods, if any, provoke an allergic reaction. The elimination/provocation technique is a four to five day period of eliminating or avoiding common food allergens. In the provocation stage, a suspected allergen is added back into the diet.

Living with Food Allergies

Figuring out which food or foods you are allergic to is just the beginning; now, you have to live the rest of your life. Some foods are easy to avoid, but the most common allergenic foods—milk, eggs, wheat, and corn—are often hidden ingredients in a myriad of processed foods. This means that, depending on the severity of your allergy, you will have to diligently scrutinize all food labels and become well versed in different names for ingredients. When eating out at restaurants, you may need to question the waiter or stick to simple dishes.

Sometimes, by carefully avoiding a food for several months or even years, you may be able to reintroduce it and no longer react to it. Another possibility is to acclimate your body to the allergenic food by eating very small amounts of the food and increasing the amount slowly. There is some evidence that this can be effective for some people to be able to tolerate foods that previously caused allergic reactions.

Lactose Intolerance

Many adults are lactose intolerant, meaning they don't produce enough of the enzyme lactase needed to digest the sugar (lactose) in dairy products. The majority of people produce lower amount of lactase as they become adults. About 25 percent of Caucasian adults of northern European descent are lactose intolerant, but 50 to 95 percent of people of other ethnic backgrounds become lactose intolerant as adults. Drinking milk or eating other dairy products will lead to stomachaches, gas, cramps, and diarrhea. These symptoms develop about thirty minutes to two hours after eating or drinking foods containing lactose.

Lactose
The sugar in milk and dairy products.

While avoiding dairy products will nip symptoms in the bud, a total avoidance may not be necessary. Many lactose intolerant people are able to tolerate certain dairy products, including yogurt, ice cream, and cheese. Supplements of lactase—the enzyme needed to digest lactose—are readily available and are taken right before a meal that contains dairy products. Lactose-reduced milk is also available.

How much lactose an intolerant person can handle varies. Thus, someone with lactose intolerance who wants to use lactase drops, capsules, or tablets, should experiment with how much she or he needs to prevent an uncomfortable reaction to milk products.

Celiac Disease—When Grains Cause Pain

Celiac disease, which is also known as celiac sprue or nontropical sprue, is a hereditary disease that occurs in about 1 out of every 5,000 Americans. It is generally diagnosed in early childhood, although it can sometimes develop after stomach surgery. People with celiac disease react to gliadin, which is found in wheat, rye, and barley. Gliadin combines with antibodies in the digestive tract and damages the walls of the small intestine. This damage interferes with the absorption of many nutrients and, if not treated, leads to malnutrition.

Gliadin
A gluten protein found in grains such as wheat, rye, and barley.

Aside from damaging the lining of the small intestine, the abnormal immune reaction to gliadin can sometimes affect other parts of the body and, in turn, increase the risk of diabetes, thyroid disease, and other health problems.

Although a few people do not have any symptoms from celiac disease, most people with this disorder suffer from frequent diarrhea, stomach upset, abdominal cramps, bloating, mouth sores, weight loss, fatigue, and slowed growth. These symptoms can range from mild to severe.

Clear, but Tough, Treatment for Celiac Disease

All gluten-containing grains (for example, wheat, barley, and rye) must be avoided in order to properly treat celiac disease. Since celiac disease is a chronic problem, a gluten-free diet must be followed closely throughout life, or else a relapse is likely. All health professionals agree upon this dietary advice. What does not have consensus of opinion is whether the additional grain, oat, should also be avoided or restricted. Oats do contain a substance similar to gliadin; however, some research has found that many people with celiac disease can eat moderate amounts of oat-containing foods without any problem. Naturally, if oats seem to cause any problems for you, it would be prudent to avoid oat-containing foods.

Gastrointestinal (GI) complaints generally resolve within a few weeks of strictly adhering to a diet completely devoid of wheat, barley, and rye and all foods containing these grains. In some cases, improvement of digestive distress, as well as improvement in nutrient absorption, might take many months.

It can be very difficult to achieve a complete avoidance of gluten because a large percentage of processed foods contain at least trace amounts of gluten, and even these trace amounts can trigger a reaction. Gluten is commonly found in prepared foods such as breads, cakes, rolls, muffins, baking mixes, pasta, breakfast cereals, beer, batter-coated foods, sauces, gravies, some soups, some candies, ice creams, and puddings. Gluten may also be hidden in foods, under such names as "cereal fillers" and "hydrolyzed protein."

If digestive problems continue after a gluten-free diet is achieved, it would be wise to look into the possibility that additional food allergies are present. Dairy foods and soy are the most likely offenders to also cause a reaction in people with celiac disease.

Restocking Nutrient Stores

The malfunctioning of the intestines that occurs with celiac disease can result in deficiencies of numerous nutrients. Even when an adequate diet is consumed, the body is simply not able to access the nutrients it needs to perform optimally. Most commonly, people with celiac disease become deficient in the minerals iron, calcium, magnesium, and zinc; the vitamins folic acid, vitamin D, and vitamin K; and the essential fatty acids.

A nutritionally minded health professional can help in the assessment for which nutrients are a problem for each individual. In the meantime, a high-potency multivitamin/mineral supplement is certainly a prudent first step. In addition, digestive enzymes in supplement form can be beneficial, particularly in the early months of treating celiac disease.

You Are What You Absorb

Sure, you've heard that "you are what you eat," but it is really more accurate to say that "you are what you absorb." You should strive to eat high-quality foods, but in order to gain the value from these foods, you need to be able to properly digest and absorb those foods. Normally, foods are digested, and then nutrients are absorbed into the bloodstream mainly from the small intestine. Malabsorption may occur either because a disorder interferes with the digestion of food or because a disorder interferes directly with the absorption of nutrients.

The most common sign that malabsorption is occurring is that a person loses weight, even though adequate amounts of food are being consumed. Diarrhea, bloating, cramping, muscle wasting, and distending abdomen can also occur. If the problem is specifically with the ability to process fats, then the stool will be light-colored, soft, and bulky and smell foul. Malabsorption can cause a deficiency of any of a number of specific vitamins, minerals, proteins, or fats, depending on the type of malabsorption problem that is present.

What Causes Malabsorption?

One cause of malabsorption is the inadequate production of digestive enzymes. Lactose intolerance is an example of this. Pancreatic enzymes are needed to digest protein and fat. If the body does not make enough of these enzymes, digestion will not be efficient.

Stomach acid production tends to decline with age; too little stomach acid can be problematic in many ways. Certain nutrients, including iron, zinc, calcium, magnesium, folic acid, and vitamin B_{12}, require stomach acid for absorption. In addition, stomach acid is needed to initiate the digestion of protein molecules.

Any disease that damages the lining of the intestine, such as celiac disease and Crohn's disease, will interfere with nutritional status, since this is where nutrients are absorbed. However, an infection such as gastroenteritis or parasitic infections with *Giardia* or another parasite can also damage the intestinal lining. Alcohol and certain drugs also have the potential to damage the lining.

An overgrowth of bacteria in the small intestine can interfere with digestion and absorption of nutrients since they can cause inflammation of the lining of the intestine.

Poor nutrient absorption happens in some cases—particularly in older or sedentary people—as the result of too little peristaltic action. This means that food that is in the process of being digested moves too slowly through the intestinal tract.

Finally, anyone who had surgery to remove part of the intestine will be at risk of nutrient deficiencies since the intestine has less surface area to process nutrients.

Absorb More Nutrients

If you have problems with nutrient absorption, the first step in getting more out of your food is to figure out the exact nature of your problem. Consultation with a health professional will be essential here. If you have a specific disease, such as celiac, Crohn's, or giardiasis, you need to know that and receive treatment.

Digestive enzymes can be helpful for some people. Enzymes are needed during the digestive process to break down food into smaller units that the body can absorb. The three classes of macronutrients in food—proteins, carbohydrates, and fats—each have a corresponding class of digestive enzymes that convert these food materials into the chemical substances used for the growth, maintenance, and repair of the body. Proteolytic enzymes (or proteases) are used for digesting protein, lipases digest fat, and amylases are needed during the digestion of carbohydrates. The pancreas produces these enzymes, which is why these three types of digestive enzymes are classified as pancreatic enzymes.

There is a spectrum of enzyme deficiencies. At the extreme end of the spectrum is the inherited condition of cystic fibrosis, in which the enzymes needed to digest proteins, carbohydrates, and fats are either missing completely or are present in only reduced amounts. Other severe conditions that are associated with enzyme deficiencies include pancreatic insufficiency, celiac disease, and Crohn's disease. The malabsorption of nutrients associated with these conditions greatly increases the risk of malnutrition. In all of the above-mentioned health problems, supplemental intake of one or more of the digestive enzymes greatly benefits health status. In addition, production of enzymes by the pancreas (both the total output and the concentration) decreases progressively with advancing age.

Tests to determine the quantity and quality of the body's production of digestive enzymes are difficult and expensive. However, it's easy to add supplemental digestive enzymes to a meal; if digestion improves, there could be an enzyme deficiency and continued supplementation would therefore be warranted.

Leaky Gut Syndrome

What would happen if your gut sprung a leak? Surprisingly, a condition known as leaky gut syndrome could play a role in health problems as diverse as Crohn's disease, celiac disease, arthritis, and asthma. The intestine plays an important balancing act. It must let in nutrients derived from food to fuel the body, but guard against the admission of waste products, bacteria, and toxins.

When the intestine is damaged for some reason—such as from nonsteroidal anti-inflammatory drugs, excessive drinking, food allergies, trauma, burns, or parasitic infection—the permeability of the intestine increases, and large, potentially harmful substances can slip through the gut barrier and into the bloodstream. These substances, in turn, trigger an immune response, and symptoms as diverse as diarrhea, rash, migraine, depression, and joint pain can occur.

Permeability
The capability to be passed through.

Leaky gut syndrome is certainly a bona-fide health condition. But whether it is common or rare continues to be a hotly debated topic among digestive health experts. What is known is that the amino acid glutamine and the mineral zinc both are vital in healing intestinal cells and, thus, tightening up a leaky gut. Even that old standby of fiber helps heal the gut to restore intestinal integrity.

Bottom Line

- The most common food allergies are to wheat, soy, dairy products, eggs, corn, citrus fruits, and nuts (including peanuts).

- The enzyme lactase is a simple fix for those unable to digest lactose in dairy products.

- People with celiac disease must completely avoid gluten from wheat and other foods; a good multivitamin/mineral supplement can help the healing process.

- Pancreatic enzymes can help if you have mal-absorption problems.

- If you have leaky gut syndrome, consider taking the amino acid glutamine and the mineral zinc.

CHAPTER 4

FEELING GREEN

While there may be the occasional person with the proverbial "iron stomach," it's pretty much a given that the rest of us will end up losing our lunch at one time or another. From motion sickness and morning sickness to the stomach flu, food poisoning, and parasites, there are a lot of hazards out there that undermine a settled stomach.

Nausea and Vomiting

There are a number of reasons that a person might feel queasy and vomit. Nausea and vomiting are very common during the first few months of pregnancy; during a bout of motion sickness when traveling by car, boat, train, or plane; as the result of an infection; after overeating; during emotional upset; or as a side effect of a medication. Gastroenteritis, which is commonly known as the "stomach flu," is another cause of nausea and vomiting.

Resting and staying hydrated are the most important things you can do to hasten recovery. Dehydration can come on very quickly when there are multiple episodes of vomiting. Even so, don't try to drink an entire glass of water at one time, since that could trigger more vomiting. Instead, take frequent small sips of a beverage, such as water, juice, or soup.

Refrain from eating until the vomiting is under

control. Until then, stick to clear liquids so that the stomach has a chance to rest and heal. When you feel up to eating, start with the BRAT diet of bland foods: Bananas, Rice, Applesauce, and Toast. When you feel hungry again—probably after about forty-eight hours—your body should be ready for more substantial foods. Even so, start with simple solid foods, such as potatoes, cooked vegetables, or eggs. Avoid dairy foods or anything fatty until you are sure that you are on the mend; these foods are difficult to digest.

Easing Queasiness

Ginger can be very useful for all manner of stomach troubles, especially nausea. It has been extensively tested for motion sickness and has been found to be more effective than Dramamine in this regard. Ginger can also be used to prevent the nausea that may develop after surgery or to reduce the queasiness and vomiting associated with chemotherapy.

Ginger also has a good track record for alleviating morning sickness in pregnant women. It is safe to use in amounts up to 1 gram daily during pregnancy. Vitamin B_6 has been recommended to alleviate morning sickness since the 1940s. Scientific studies continue to confirm that vitamin B_6 can help some women have fewer episodes of vomiting.

Food Poisoning

Unless you are a tyrant ruling a contested kingdom, food poisoning is not as exciting as it might sound. In fact, it is as unexciting, in most cases, as food being handled by unwashed hands.

Food poisoning is one of the most common infections, following just behind the common cold. There are more than 200 diseases that can be spread through contaminated food, with the most common infectious organisms being *Salmonella, E. coli, Listeria, Clostridium, Staphylococcus aureus,* and *Trichinella.* About 20 percent of the time, the faulty handling or preparation of the food in question happens at home, and almost 80 percent of the time, it is traced to a food-service outlet.

Food poisoning causes nausea, vomiting, diarrhea, abdominal pain and cramping, fever, and general malaise. Food poisoning is often mistaken for the stomach flu.

Prevention of Food Poisoning Is Your Best Bet

Foods of animal origin are most susceptible to contamination. The infectious agent can be introduced, or allowed to grow, as a result of unwashed hands preparing the food, meat not being cooked long enough or at a high enough temperature, foods being left out of refrigeration too long, being canned improperly, or cross contamination, such as when a cutting board is used for raw meat and then vegetables.

Minor food-poisoning episodes can usually be treated at home with rest and prevention of dehydration, caused by the vomiting or diarrhea. As unpleasant as the vomiting and diarrhea are, it is best to let nature run its course to rid the body of the harmful organisms. Sip on water, diluted juice, or weak tea to stay hydrated. Ginger tea is a good choice since it helps quell nausea. Green tea is another good option since it has antibacterial and immune-boosting properties.

Don't tax your digestive system with food again until you feel up to it. Reintroduce foods gradually, with easily digested foods such as toast, applesauce, bananas, rice, or diluted juices. When you are on the road to recovery, you might consider taking a probiotic supplement to rein-troduce beneficial flora to your gut.

Are You Hosting Parasites?

Parasites are far less common than in the past, thanks to improvements in sanitation and living conditions. In fact, some parasitic infections that were once ubiquitous have all but disappeared from developed countries with clean water and reliable food supplies. However, a few parasites have proven themselves to be resistant, and others are even becoming more prevalent as in-ternational travel becomes more popular. Infes-tations with parasites are also more common in children, those who live in institutional settings, and anyone with a compromised immune sys-tem. The most likely parasites to be living in you are *Giardia, Entamoeba histolytica, Cryptospor-idium*, roundworm, hookworm, pinworm, and tapeworm.

Intestinal parasites come in a wide variety of shapes and sizes, but the majority are either sin-gle-celled protozoa or worms. Regardless of their appearance, all of these parasites survive by feeding on the cells and tissues of the host. There is a long list of problems that parasites can cause for the host, such as fever, anemia, gas, bloating, diarrhea, constipation, loss of appetite and weight loss, abdominal cramps and pain, nausea, vomiting, rash, itching anus, and bloody or foul-smelling stools.

It can be very difficult to get an accurate diag-nosis of parasitic infection since the symptoms are similar to so many other health conditions, and many times physicians don't think of the possibility.

Sidestep Unwelcome Bacteria

Basic hygiene rules—the same ones your mom

drilled into you—are still the best way to stay healthy. First and foremost, it is important to wash your hands every time you use the bathroom and before eating.

If you are traveling in developing countries, it is very important to not drink the local water from the tap, and to avoid uncooked foods, street vendor foods, ice, and fruits that aren't able to be peeled. Within your own country, there are also ways to protect yourself, such as never drinking untreated stream water while camping and thoroughly cooking fish, meat, and poultry. Apologies to those who love steak tartare, sushi, and raw oysters, but consuming these foods is just not a good idea.

Pets can also be a source of parasitic infection, specifically worms. Animal feces can contaminate soil in parks and playgrounds with eggs, and children can easily get infected this way. Again, hand washing cannot be stressed more strongly. Don't let animals lick you on the mouth, keep your pet free of fleas, and be meticulous about cleaning up any "accidents" in the house.

Can Herbs Boot Out Parasites?

Conventional medicine turns to some serious medications to eradicate parasites; unfortunately, these drugs, such as metronidazole (Flagyl), can also cause quite a few discomforts for the host. There are herbs that have parasite-fighting credentials, but they are in the same boat as the medications—that is, used in the strong doses needed to kill the parasites can also leave you vulnerable to some side effects, such as stomach upset, intestinal cramps, or liver damage. In any event, when facing down parasites, you'd be best served by working with an herbalist or other health professional for diagnosis and treatment, rather than self-treating at home.

In the laboratory, garlic has been shown to kill parasites, but human research hasn't been done yet. It certainly wouldn't hurt to flavor your food liberally with garlic if you are infected with parasites and pursuing treatment. While you're at it, you might snack on some handfuls of pumpkin seeds—they also have purported parasite-fighting action.

A compound called berberine is found in several plants that have yellow roots, including goldenseal, goldthread, barberry, and Oregon grape. It has been found to successfully treat giardia. However, this is one of the cases in which the high levels needed for success could potentially cause side effects. Therefore, it should only be used with the guidance of a health professional.

Bottom Line

- Ginger is the premier herb to quell queasiness.

- Prevention is best for food poisoning; if it's too late for prevention, you might sip on green tea or ginger tea and pamper your GI tract with some probiotics.

- Parasites are best treated with the help of a health professional rather than at home. Garlic, pumpkin seeds, or berberine-containing herbs might be recommended by a health professional.

CHAPTER 5

DIGESTION-RELATED ORGANS: LIVER AND GALLBLADDER

There are a wide variety of health problems that can afflict internal organs related to digestion. The ones covered in this chapter include gallbladder disease, liver disease, and hiatal hernia.

Gallstone Basics

Gallstones are round lumps of solid matter (often cholesterol) found in the gallbladder and sometimes in the bile ducts. These lumps form when the liquid bile that is stored in the gallbladder hardens into pieces of stonelike material. Gallstones can be as tiny as a grain of sand or as large as a golf ball. Just one large stone, hundreds of tiny stones, or almost any combination of stones can develop in the gallbladder.

Bile
Liquid that is made in the liver and then stored in the gallbladder until needed by the body to help digest fats.

Bile is made of cholesterol, fats, bile salts, proteins, and bilirubin. If the bile contains some of these constituents in the wrong proportions, a stone is more likely to form. Eighty percent of gallstones are cholesterol stones, primarily made of hardened cholesterol. The rest are pigment stones; they are made of bilirubin, the substance in bile that gives it, as well as stool, a yellowish color.

Problems arise when gallstones lodge in any of the ducts that carry bile from the liver to the small intestine and block the normal flow of bile. Bile then becomes trapped in these ducts and can cause inflammation in the gallbladder, the ducts themselves, or even the liver.

A gallstone attack is very painful, with the pain located in the upper-right quarter of the abdomen, and often wrapping around to the back. Nausea and vomiting can also occur. Gallstone attacks often occur after eating a meal. Symptoms can mimic those of other problems, including a heart attack.

Who Gets Gallstones?

Gallstones are much more common than many people realize, since they only cause noticeable problems about 20 percent of the time. Gallstones occur more often in women than in men; in fact, they are two to three times more likely to crop up in women. High estrogen levels, as a result of pregnancy, hormone replacement therapy, or birth control pills, can increase the amount of cholesterol in bile and lead to gallstones.

Being overweight is a major risk factor for gallstones, particularly in women. The prevailing theory accounting for this is that obesity tends to lower the amount of bile salts in bile, which increases the proportion of cholesterol. Excess weight also slows emptying of the gallbladder. Losing weight lowers the risk of gallstones, but ironically, losing weight too fast can also up the chances of forming a gallstone because the fat that is metabolized causes the liver to send extra cholesterol into bile.

High rates of gallstones are also seen in adults over age sixty, Native Americans, Mexican Amer- icans, diabetics, and anyone on cholesterol-lowering drugs.

If you tend toward being constipated and have gallstones, you'd probably benefit from resolving your constipation. Refer to Chapter 2 for advice on treating constipation.

Dietary Advice for Gallstone Formers

Since cholesterol is the main constituent of 80 percent of gallstones, consuming less cholesterol can be a good idea. Coffee drinking is actually a helpful thing, since coffee boosts the flow of bile. The caffeine in coffee is responsible for the benefit, since people drinking decaffeinated coffee were not found to have a lower risk of gallstones.

Plant proteins in general, and soy protein, in particular, have been shown to prevent gallstones. And soy may even shrink a gallstone after it has developed. Vegetarians, who often include frequent servings of soy in their diets, suffer from only half the gallstones of nonvegetarians.

Food allergies are not a cause of forming stones, but might trigger a gallbladder attack in someone who has stones. If you think that food allergies might play a role in your attacks, take a look at Chapter 3 to find out more about food allergies.

The herb milk thistle might help prevent gallstones from forming. Milk thistle extract containing the active component silymarin lowers the amount of cholesterol in bile. Another helpful supplement is phosphatidylcholine, which helps prevent gallstone formation and may even dissolve existing stones.

Vitamin C is another supplement to consider, since this vitamin might lessen stone formation by converting cholesterol to bile acids.

The Amazing Liver

The liver is a very important organ that performs thousands of vital chemical and metabolic functions, including the storage of fat-soluble vitamins, iron, and glycogen (a form of carbohydrate) for when the body needs these nutrients at a later date. In addition, it makes cholesterol and amino acids, removes wastes from the blood, detoxifies alcohol and other toxins, and breaks down most medications.

Unlike most other organs, the liver can regenerate itself. Even so, it can be damaged severely by disease or toxins beyond the point of repair. Alcohol is the leading cause of liver disease, often leading to the liver disease cirrhosis. The scarring in the liver caused by cirrhosis is irreversible. As with all liver problems, stopping drinking alcohol is essential to preventing further damage. After cirrhosis, hepatitis is the next most common liver disease. There are many different types of hepatitis, and unfortunately, there are not a lot of conventional treatment options for any of them, aside from rest and avoidance of alcohol.

Eating to Be Kind to the Liver

Anyone with liver disease should choose a diet that is the least burdensome to the liver. This means absolutely no alcohol, minimizing fatty foods, and eating only small amounts of protein (about two ounces a day). Proteins from plant sources, such as grains and le-gumes, are easier for the liver to handle than animal source proteins. A low-salt diet and plenty of fluids are also important.

Cirrhosis
Liver disease in which healthy liver cells are replaced by scar tissue, which prevents it from functioning normally.

The herb milk thistle has the remarkable ability to protect the liver from damage as well as stimulate the growth of new, healthy liver cells. This is the herb of choice for all variety of liver problems. In fact, milk thistle has been used as a liver remedy for more than 2,000 years. A compound in milk thistle called silymarin is the active constituent; check for herb extracts that are standardized to contain high levels (such as 80 percent) of this compound.

Please note, if you choose to take herbs when you have liver problems, do not take herbal tinctures, as these contain alcohol.

Phospholipids, and especially phosphatidylcholine, are normal constituents of cell membranes, which carry out practically all of the functions of the liver. Scientific studies demonstrate that phosphatidylcholine has a restoring effect on the liver and actually assists the liver in recovery from toxic attack, such as from the toxins in tobacco, alcohol, certain mushrooms, viruses, and over-the-counter and pharmaceutical drugs. Overall, phosphatidylcholine has been shown to prevent and even reverse liver damage.

Phospholipids
Family of fat-soluble compounds that are needed in cell membranes.

What Is a Hiatal Hernia?

Hiatal hernia, a condition in which the opening where the esophagus and stomach meet becomes overly wide and protrudes, is a common cause of recurring indigestion. Some hiatal hernias are present at birth; however, most develop later in life as the opening (hiatus) becomes stretched as a result of pregnancy or obesity—both of which place upward pressure on the stomach. Coughing, vomiting, and straining during bowel movements can also stretch the hiatus.

Hiatus
The small opening in the diaphragm where the esophagus meets the stomach.

For those over age fifty, the chances that a hiatal hernia is present are better than fifty-fifty. Most people, however, are unaware of the hernia because it is minor enough to not cause any symptoms. For those who do experience symptoms, the list of discomforts is topped by heartburn, since the stretched out opening allows stomach acid to cause a burning sensation in the esophagus. Even so, this is not generally a serious problem, unless the frequent exposure to stomach acids damages the esophagus.

Treating Hiatal Hernias

Treating a hiatal hernia can be as simple as not wearing constrictive clothing and losing excess weight so that the pressure is lessened on the stomach. Many of the same tips that help heartburn (discussed in Chapter 1), apply here, such as avoiding large meals and instead eating four or five smaller meals throughout the day. Do not eat or drink anything for at least two hours before bed, and stay upright for at least an hour after eating.

Avoiding alcohol, coffee, tobacco, fatty foods, and any foods that you notice provoke indigestion makes sense. If you have constipation, see Chapter 2 for tips on how to treat it so that you aren't straining during bowel movements and worsening your hiatal hernia. If you often have symptoms of your hiatal hernia at night, you might try raising the head of your bed three to six inches to help keep your stomach in place and prevent reflux of stomach acid.

Bottom Line

- Milk thistle and phosphatidylcholine are both potentially beneficial for the treatment of gallstones, as well as for enhancing overall liver health.

- For any manner of liver problem, it is essential to avoid alcohol, to eat a low-fat diet, and to choose plant proteins in place of animal sources of protein.

- Hiatal hernias are treated in much the same way as indigestion—such as eating smaller meals, avoiding fatty foods, and avoiding alcohol.

CHAPTER 6

CANCER OF THE DIGESTIVE SYSTEM

Do you think that there's not much you can do about your risk of cancer? Think again. Diet is estimated to contribute to about one-third of preventable cancers—about the same amount as smoking. Not surprisingly, the foods that you eat tend to have the biggest impact on cancers of the digestive tract. For someone who will develop cancer this year, there is a one in five chance that it will be in the digestive system, such as the colon/rectum or stomach.

Sensible Approach to Preventing Cancer

Cancer prevention is based on many of the same recommendations that promote overall health: don't use tobacco and avoid exposure to secondhand smoke, limit sun exposure, and avoid chemicals in the environment. The following are also tried-and-true tips for minimizing your risk of cancer:

- Eat a variety of healthful foods, with an emphasis on plant sources.

- Eat five or more servings of a variety of vegetables and fruits every day.

- Choose whole grains instead of refined grains and sugars (such as white flour and white rice) found in processed foods .

- Limit consumption of red meats, especially those high in fat, and processed meats such as bacon and luncheon meats.

- Maintain a healthy body weight.

- Engage in physical activity, with the goal being at least thirty minutes a day, five times a week.

- If you drink alcoholic beverages, limit your consumption.

Anticancer Food and Drinks

The stomach and other parts of the digestive system are the frontlines when it comes to exposure to cancer-promoters in foods—but anticancer substances in food can also exert a strong effect here. Take garlic. The potential of garlic as a cancer fighter has been known since ancient times. However, scientific research documenting the anticancer ability of garlic wasn't available until the 1930s. At that time, scientists charted the occurrence of cancer in countries with varied garlic intakes. They discovered that cancer cases were least common in the countries with the highest garlic consumption.

Human studies of garlic and cancer have been very promising. For example, stomach cancer risk drops by up to 40 percent in people eating large amounts of garlic and onions. A study of 41,000 women in Iowa found that eating garlic at least once a week reduced the risk of colon cancer by 35 percent.

Garlic is a great addition to many dishes, although a few people might be sensitive to garlic and experience heartburn after indulging. And for those with a sensitive nose, it's good to know that odor-controlled supplements of garlic are on the market. Note: people who take anticlotting drugs should talk to their doctors before taking garlic supplements, since garlic has blood-thinning qualities.

Just about any way you pour it, tea is great for your health. Green tea sets the standard for health protection, since this light and tasty tea has the highest levels of a type of antioxidant called polyphenols. Numerous research studies link a high intake of green tea to a lower risk of various cancers.

But black tea is no slouch, either. For instance, when the tea-drinking habits of 35,369 American women were compared to their incidence of cancer over an eight-year period, the women who regularly drank tea (primarily black tea, which also contains the healthful polyphenols) showed a lower risk of cancers of the upper digestive tract.

While you're pouring a beverage to go with your meal, you might want to consider red wine, which is another rich source of polyphenols, as well as other cancer-fighting nutrients. It can be a balancing act, however. Alcohol in general is linked to the promotion of cancer, but if you are going to drink an alcoholic beverage, red wine has cancer-fighting properties.

Polyphenols
A family of antioxidants found in plants.

The evidence on whether dietary fiber exerts a protective role in reducing the incidence of colorectal cancer is mixed. However, considering that fiber has many beneficial roles in healthy digestive function, there is no reason not to err on the side of consuming a fiber-rich diet.

Researchers report a consistent pattern of cancer protection when even small amounts of fish are included in a person's diet on a regular basis. Fish contains a type of essential fatty acid called omega-3s (specifically EPA and DHA). Superior sources of omega-3s include salmon, herring, sardines, cod, tuna, and mackerel. If fish aren't to your liking, flaxseed oil is another source of omega-3s. Fish oil supplements are also an option, although some people may experience a little stomach upset from these pills. It's also a good idea to pop some extra vitamin E (about 200 IU) when taking fish oil supplements, since fish oil is easily attacked by free radicals.

Cancer-Promoting Foods

It cuts both ways: Just as certain foods can stymie cancer cells from growing in the first place, other foods can provide fertile ground for cancer growth. This doesn't mean that you can never have foods that contain these ingredients, but it is prudent to use them in moderation. For example, food additives called nitrites, found in processed meats such as bacon and bologna, are converted in the body to nitrosamines, which are potent carcinogens. Other dietary mutagens include aflatoxin (a mold that forms on peanuts), heavy metals such as lead, polychlorinated biphenyls (PCBs), and pesticides such as malathione and DDT. Alcohol does not initiate cancer, but it promotes the growth of existing abnormal cells. Other suspected dietary promoters are saccharine, saturated fat, trans fatty acids, and caffeine.

Natural Cancer Fighters

When it comes to the health of your body's cells, public enemy number one are free radicals. These dangerous rogues react with just about any molecule in the body, including fats, proteins, or even DNA within cells. And when areas of damaged DNA accumulate, cancer can be the scary consequence.

Fortunately, your body is prepared with an antioxidant defense system. Antioxidants, such as vitamins A, C, and E, and other nutrients and enzymes, neutralize free radicals to preserve healthy cells. Fruits and vegetables are chock-full with potent antioxidants, and boosting consumption of these foods is a widely accepted way to lower the risk of most common cancers.

If dodging cancer is important to you, you'll want to make sure you're getting enough folic acid. Diminished folic acid status has been linked to an increased risk of cancers of the colon and other organs. Good food sources of folic acid include dark green leafy vegetables, orange juice, and broccoli. Folic acid is also found in multivitamin supplements, B-complex supplements, and even as stand-alone supplements.

It is thought that calcium lowers colon cancer risk by binding bile acids and fatty acids, thereby reducing exposure in the large intestine to toxic compounds. Numerous studies have found an inverse relationship between calcium intake and cancer risk.

Over the past few years, selenium has gained solid foothold as a cancer preventive agent. Selenium is thought to reduce the risk of cancer through its role in the production of the antioxidant en - zyme glutathione peroxidase—an enzyme that guards against free-radical damage within cells.

There are several studies linking selenium to cancer prevention, including a double-blind trial involving more than 1,300 individuals that reported a clear drop in cancer death rate in men taking 200 mcg of yeast-based selenium daily for four and a half years compared with the placebo (sugar pill) group. The body more readily uses the natural yeast form of selenium than the selenite form of selenium.

Helpful Bacteria in the Gut

Research spanning several decades suggests that friendly bacteria may help prevent cancer.

Probiotics reduce the risk of colon cancer by changing the pH of the colon and by isolating cancer-causing substances so that they can be excreted. In addition, probiotics, by helping to maintain regular bowel movements, prevent carcinogens in waste matter from staying too long in the lower intestine and attacking normal cells. Probiotics also suppress tumor cells, inhibit bacteria that produce cancer-causing enzymes, and deactivate carcinogenic substances called nitrosamines.

pH
A measure of acidity.

Bottom Line

- Diet can both contribute to and provide protection from digestive system cancers.

- Top nutritional factors that bolster resistance to cancers of the stomach, colon, and rectum include garlic, green tea, fish oil, antioxidants (vitamins A, C, and E), folic acid, calcium, selenium, and probiotics.

CHAPTER 7

PROTECTING THE STOMACH'S LINING

The lining of the stomach has a very important role. It protects the delicate tissue underneath from the corrosive action of stomach acid. Anytime the stomach lining is compromised, such as in gastritis and peptic ulcer, pain and other symptoms are sure to arise.

Peptic Ulcer

An ulcer is any sore on the body, but when someone says that they have an ulcer, they almost always mean a "peptic" ulcer. Peptic ulcers develop when the mucous membrane lining the stomach or the duodenum is eroded and is no longer able to protect the tissue below. Peptic

Duodenum
The upper portion of the intestines, directly below the stomach.

ulcers are quite common, with about one in every ten adults having one at some point in life. Men are four times more likely than women to have an ulcer.

Occasionally, a peptic ulcer can be painless, but in most people, the pain is the primary symptom. It tends to be a dull, gnawing ache in the upper abdomen that develops a few hours after a meal or in the middle of the night (when the stomach is empty). The pain can come and go for several days or weeks. Eating can ease the discomfort. Peptic ulcers can also cause weight loss, poor appetite, bloating, burping, nausea, and vomiting. Untreated ulcers often bleed.

What Causes an Ulcer?

For many years, stress and spicy foods were thought to be at the root of peptic ulcers. Today, both of these suspects are off the hook (although stress and diet can certainly aggravate an existing ulcer). The real culprit of most ulcers is the bacterium *Helicobacter pylori* (*H. pylori*). This bacterium was discovered in 1982, when researchers found that antibiotics can destroy *H. pylori* and cure peptic ulcers. Other ulcers can be caused by use of nonsteroidal anti-inflammatory agents (NSAIDs), like aspirin and ibuprofen. These drugs should be avoided by anyone with peptic ulcers. Occasionally, cancerous tumors in the stomach or pancreas can cause ulcers.

Infection with *H. pylori* is quite common, with about 20 percent of people under age forty and 50 percent of those over age sixty having it. Fortunately, just having the bacteria does not mean that an ulcer is inevitable—most infected people, in fact, do not develop ulcers. It is not yet known what other factors cause *H. pylori* to trigger an ulcer. It is known, however, that *H. pylori* is able to weaken the protective mucous membrane that lines the stomach and duodenum, thus allowing the damaging stomach acid to reach the sensitive tissue beneath to cause an ulcer. *H. pylori* is also known to increase the risk of stomach cancer.

Helicobacter pylori
The only germ hardy enough to survive the acidic stomach environment; infection with it can lead to an ulcer.

A combination of antibiotics and bismuth (such as Pepto-Bismol) is the typical treatment for peptic ulcers. You can also give dietary changes and a handful of supplements a try. These are discussed in the following sections.

Be Kind to Your Stomach

A completely bland diet was once *de rigueur* for anyone with an ulcer, but now that *H. pylori,* as opposed to spicy foods, is known to cause ulcers, the thinking on this has changed. Even so, if you notice that certain spicy foods, or any other particular foods, worsen your ulcer, it makes sense to avoid them. There is some evidence that food allergies might play a role in peptic ulcers. Thus, it might be helpful to determine if food allergies are present and avoid those foods (see Chapter 3).

Salty foods can irritate the stomach, and it would be prudent to restrict the use of salt. Likewise, alcohol, coffee (caffeinated as well as decaf), and tea should also be avoided.

Cabbage juice can help heal peptic ulcers, but quite a bit of it needs to be consumed. The research with this unusual beverage found that drinking a quart a day of cabbage juice for up to two weeks might relieve symptoms of peptic ulcers. Eating a diet that is high in fiber is an - other smart choice to help prevent the recurrence of ulcers.

Natural Ulcer Healers

Although the herb licorice shares the same name as the child's candy, it is rarely the same substance. The herb licorice used to be used to flavor candy, but today, most "licorice" candy is flavored with anise. Even if real licorice candy can be found, it contains too little licorice to be used as an herbal remedy. Instead, licorice products that are labeled as an herbal remedy should be used. Licorice root is very soothing to the mucous membranes of the GI tract, and even ups the stomach's output of mucin—the key substance in stomach lining that blocks the corrosion of stomach acid.

The only downside to licorice root is that it contains a compound called glycyrrhizin that can increase blood pressure and cause water retention. Ordinary licorice should not be taken for more than ten days in a row. Fortunately, there is a slightly processed form of the herb called deglycyrrhizinated licorice (DGL) that has removed the troublesome compound, while leaving behind the stomach-friendly parts. DGL has been shown to speed the healing of ulcers. The chewable tablets are preferable to the capsules.

Additional herbs that have a soothing effect on irritated mucous membranes are chamomile and marshmallow. Ayurvedic medicine has often turned to dried banana powder to heal ulcers. Research, in both animals and humans, confirms that dried banana helps cases of peptic ulcer. It is not yet known if simply eating bananas could have the same beneficial effect.

Ayurvedic Medicine
A 5,000-year-old system of healing developed in India. It combines natural therapies, such as herbs, with a personalized approach to the treatment of disease.

Vitamin A and the mineral zinc are both important during the healing process of the stomach lining. It should be noted, however, that pregnant women should not take more than 10,000 IU per day of vitamin A. Another nutrient that can be useful for the healing process of the intestinal lining and stomach is an amino acid called glutamine. Although the original research with glutamine and peptic ulcers is several decades old and has yet to be followed up, it could be helpful to take up to 1,000 mg of glutamine per day during the acute phase of a peptic ulcer.

Finally, you might consider the herb garlic for getting to the source of the problem. In the laboratory, garlic has been shown to inhibit the growth of *H. pylori*. Unfortunately, follow-up research with people afflicted with *H. pylori* infections did not show the garlic to be successful in destroying the infection.

Gastritis: Peptic Ulcer's Cousin

Gastritis is a general term for inflammation that affects the stomach lining. It can arise as a result of an infection (including by *H. pylori*), excessive use of aspirin or other nonsteroidal anti-inflammatory drugs, a disease such as Crohn's, or even physical stress such as the flu, surgery, or burns. Alcohol and tobacco use can also be causative factors. In some people, gastritis may cause no symptoms, even as it erodes the stomach lining and causes internal bleeding. Others may develop abdominal pain, indigestion, nausea, and belching as a result of the gastritis.

For many people, gastritis is the first step on the road to an ulcer. Not surprisingly, all of the advice given previously in this chapter about preventing and treating peptic ulcers applies to gastritis, as well. For starters—like with peptic ulcers—eliminating *H. pylori* infection is important. The accepted way to do this is with antibiotics and bismuth medication.

As with peptic ulcers, it is prudent to limit salt and caffeine intake as well as ferreting out any potential food allergies.

In addition to the herbs, vitamins, and minerals that were discussed for treating peptic ulcer, people with gastritis might also benefit from taking a supplement called gamma-oryzanol. Gamma-oryzanol is a mixture of plant compounds called sterols and ferulic acid esters found in rice bran, corn, and barley oils. Several trials have put this supplement to the test in people with gastritis with very promising results.

Bottom Line

- Ulcers can respond well to DGL licorice, chamomile, marshmallow, banana powder, vitamin A, zinc, glutamine, or garlic.

- If you have gastritis, all of the supplements that are useful for ulcers can help, as well as gamma-oryzanol.

CHAPTER 8

INFLAMMATORY BOWEL DISEASE: CROHN'S DISEASE AND ULCERATIVE COLITIS

One million Americans know the pain of inflammatory bowel disease—an umbrella term for Crohn's disease and ulcerative colitis. Both of these conditions cause inflammation of the intestines, but the difference is that ulcerative colitis affects only the colon and rectum, while Crohn's disease—the more serious of the two—involves more extensive areas of the intestines.

Crohn's Disease on the Rise

Inflammatory bowel diseases are growing at a rate that has both alarmed and baffled doctors. Crohn's disease, named after the doctor who first identified the disease in the 1930s, doubled in occurrence between then and 1970, and its incidence has subsequently tripled. This sharp increase is particularly vexing since the most common victim is in the prime of his or her life (that is, ages twenty to forty). The hallmark signs of Crohn's are chronic diarrhea, abdominal cramps and pain, a low-grade fever, fatigue, and weight loss. It can seem as though food has turned against you, since the episodes of pain and diarrhea, which can be quite severe and debilitating, generally follow mealtime.

What could be fueling this epidemic? Experts are still unclear about the specifics, but they do know that there is something in our Western lifestyle that must be the culprit since the highest concentration of new cases are in Western countries. What is known is that having a relative with Crohn's disease can put you at ten times greater risk of developing the disease yourself, and if that relative is a sibling, then your risk jumps thirty times greater than average. Aside from this genetic link, Crohn's disease seems to be triggered by something in the environment (perhaps a bacteria or virus) that sets off an abnormal immune response.

The really bad news is that Crohn's disease has no cure, and the standard treatments can often impair quality of life as much as the disease itself. Drugs such as steroids, aspirinlike medications, and immune suppressants are among the standard arsenal. Almost 75 percent of people with Crohn's disease end up having surgery to remove inflamed areas of intestine or deal with related complications of the disease, such as blockage, perforation, or intestinal bleeding. However, even this drastic measure is not a long-term fix since the disease recurs in almost all cases.

Making Friends with Food Again

Good nutrition and dietary supplements play important roles in Crohn's disease. First, they can prolong periods of remission. And second, they can provide some relief of symptoms during an active episode of the disease.

Food allergies appear to be involved. Many people report that their disease flares up when certain trigger foods are eaten. Which foods act as triggers is particular to each individual; however, spicy foods, high-fiber foods, milk, and alcohol are common culprits. It's worth the time to sleuth out which foods could be setting you off.

Deficiencies of numerous vitamins and minerals are common in those with Crohn's disease, in large part due to the chronic diarrhea that flushes away nutrients before the body can use them. A multivitamin/mineral supplement can provide some measure of protection against deficiencies.

Zinc, folic acid, and vitamin B_{12} are among the most common deficiencies. For the person with Crohn's disease, not having enough of these nutrients is like adding fuel to a raging fire since these nutrients are needed by the body to repair damaged intestinal cells. Zinc has another important role in the gut—that of maintaining proper permeability. The healthy GI tract strikes just the right balance between letting molecules of food in and keeping out bacteria and toxins. In the case of a "leaky gut," this balance is tipped in favor of just about any molecule (healthy or not) that happens by. One study of Crohn's disease patients currently in remission found that zinc supplements tightened up the leaky gut and helped prevent future episodes of Crohn's disease.

A particular species of probiotic bacteria called *lactobacillus GG* has been studied in children with Crohn's disease and has been found to both aid the healing of a leaky gut as well as improve overall disease activity. Another species of bacteria, called *Saccharomyces boulardii* can be helpful in lessening chronic diarrhea, as well as prolonging remission times.

Fishing for a Way to Feel Better

Fish is a natural anti-inflammatory. Not surprising, then, is the very low occurrence of Crohn's disease in traditional fish-eating Eskimo populations. The omega-3 fatty acids found in fish oil are the real star when it comes to quelling inflammation. Supplements of the omega-3 fatty acids EPA and DHA can be a great aid in prolonging the time between flare-ups. For many people, fish oil supplements taken in the high amounts needed to garner benefits (generally several grams daily) can cause side effects of bad breath, "fishy" burps, and even diarrhea. Fortunately, there is a special enteric-coated "free fatty acid" form of EPA/DHA available that has been documented in double-blind research to reduce the recurrence rate of Crohn's disease without the troublesome side effects.

Gut-Friendly Herbs

A handful of herbs can help soothe an inflamed digestive tract. These comforting botanicals include marshmallow, slippery elm, chamomile, and licorice. If you're in the grip of a flare-up of diarrhea, tannin-containing herbs (such as green tea) can provide a small measure of relief. But keep in mind that you should stop taking these herbs as the diarrhea lets up; otherwise, they could actually aggravate your condition.

Peppermint oil is best known for treating IBS, but since the symptoms of this problem are similar to Crohn's disease (in fact, many Crohn's sufferers are misdiagnosed with IBS), it makes sense that peppermint oil might help in Crohn's disease. Although there are no formal studies yet, you can give enteric-coated peppermint oil capsules a try to ease abdominal cramps and pain. Some people can't tolerate these capsules, however, as they sometimes cause heartburn or other GI upset.

Bottom Line

- Inflammatory bowel disease can lead to deficiencies of zinc, folic acid, and vitamin B_{12}.

- Probiotics and "free fatty acid" fish oil (EPA/DHA) can help prevent recurrences of these diseases.

- Helpful herbs for these conditions include marshmallow, slippery elm, chamomile, green tea, and peppermint oil.

CHAPTER 9

THE FINAL STOP

G iven that the colon/rectum is the end of the line in food's journey through the digestive tract, it is fitting that the final chapter of this book is devoted to colorectal health concerns. Diverticulitis, hemorrhoids, and gas are among the more common afflictions. In addition, this chapter provides information about enemas and other forms of colon therapy and discusses the importance of bacteria that make their home in the colon.

Diverticulitis

When small pouches (called diverticula) protrude from the wall of the colon, the stage is set for the disease of diverticulitis. The pouches themselves are not a problem, but they can easily become filled with the waste material that is flowing through the large intestines. If this waste sits in the pouch for too long, it can become infected.

Diverticulitis most often hits after age sixty, in people who are overweight, and—most impor-tant—in those with a low-fiber diet. The suspect-ed sequence of events goes like this: too little fiber and water in the diet creates small, hard, dry stools that are difficult to pass. The straining that then occurs during bowel movements puts pres-sure on the intestinal walls. Areas that are weak-ened by this constant straining balloon outward to form a pouch. These pouches are thought to occur in 50 percent of Americans by age sixty and nearly all by age eighty. Fortunately, only a small percentage of those with pouches will develop an infection and have symptoms.

Abdominal cramps and pain, gas, fever, rectal bleeding, constipation, and diarrhea are all common symptoms of this disease. Serious complications, such as abscesses, intestinal obstructions, or perforations of the intestinal wall can develop.

Fiber, Fiber, and More Fiber

Too little fiber is the leading dietary cause of diverticulitis, and fiber is the solution. A diet rich in fruits and vegetables helps prevent the development of diverticulitis. Not surprisingly, vegetarians are much less likely to have this disease. If you currently have a low-fiber diet, you'll want to transition slowly to a high-fiber diet, since a sudden change can upset the digestive tract. In addition, it is very important to increase fluid intake when increasing your intake of fiber so that the stool remains soft and moves easily through the digestive tract.

Since constipation contributes to diverticulitis, it is important to improve your regularity. Refer to Chapter 2 for constipation remedies that can also help with diverticulitis, such as psyllium and glucomannan.

If you have diverticulitis, avoid foods that have small, hard particles that can become lodged in the pouches, such as seeds, nuts, hulls, or strings. Instead, choose whole-grain cereals, breads, and seedless fruits and vegetables.

A few select herbs can help soothe an intestine inflamed with diverticulitis. Chamomile and peppermint are premier in this area.

Hemorrhoids

Hemorrhoids are one of the most common ailments known, with more than half the population experiencing them at some point in life. Hemorrhoids are varicose veins that occur in the anus and rectum. In general, they are the result of excessive pressure on the veins of the anus and rectum. They are more common with advancing age, during pregnancy, and if you have a family history, experience frequent constipation or diarrhea, or overuse laxatives or enemas.

Varicose Veins
Enlarged, bulging blood vessels.

Hemorrhoids are classified as either internal or external, depending on their location. External hemorrhoids feel like a hard lump and are very sensitive. Internal hemorrhoids can protrude during bowel movements, which may or may not be painful. Other symptoms of hemorrhoids are itching in the anal area or bleeding during bowel movements.

Hemorrhoids are not linked to a higher risk of cancer; however, the symptom of bleeding can also be a sign of colorectal cancer and should therefore be ruled out by a physician.

How Are Hemorrhoids Treated?

The straining that accompanies constipation places undo pressure on the veins of that area, either causing or worsening hemorrhoids. Therefore, treating underlying constipation is an important first step for resolving hemorrhoids. Take a look at Chapter 2 for detailed information about how to treat constipation.

As with most problems of the lower digestive tract, increasing your fiber intake is a helpful place to start. People who have a higher fiber intake are less likely to develop hemorrhoids. Remember to drink more fluids any time you eat more fiber. The insoluble form of fiber, which is primarily found in whole grains and vegetables, makes the stool softer, bulkier, and easier to pass. Supplemental fibers, such as psyllium seeds, can also be used to increase fiber intake.

In the meantime, sitting in a warm sitz bath can help relieve the pain and itching of hemorrhoids. The herb witch hazel has astringent properties that can help shrink hemorrhoids. It can be applied as an ointment to the affected area a few times a day. A gel containing the herb horse chestnut extract can be used for the same purpose.

Vitamin C and a class of nutrients called flavonoids help heal and strengthen blood vessels. Eating more fruits and vegetables to up your fiber intake will naturally provide more of these nutrients, as well. They are also available as supplements.

Passing Gas

Everyone has gas. Burping or passing gas is normal, but because it is embarrassing or uncomfortable, many people worry that they have an abnormal amount. The average person will pass gas more than a dozen times a day, most of which isn't noticed. It's only when excessive amounts of gas build up, leading to a bloated, painful feeling or when the gas is malodorous that it becomes problematic. Most of the time gas is odorless. The odor comes from sulfur made by bacteria in the large intestine. In addition to the digestive process, air can be swallowed while eating or drinking, and add to the amount of gas in the intestinal tract.

Flatulence becomes more common with age, and some people just seem more susceptible to gassy episodes than others. Some basic tips that can be helpful include the following:

- Eat smaller portions.

- Chew food thoroughly.

- Sip, rather than gulp, liquids.

- Avoid carbonated beverages.

- Do not chew gum.

- Do not drink with a straw.

- Remain in an upright position while eating.

- The product Beano contains natural enzymes that reduce gas when it is used along with troublesome foods.

Foods to Eat, Foods to Avoid

Certain foods are notorious gas producers. Beans and legumes, in particular, can cause foul-smelling gas for many people. Soaking beans overnight and then discarding this water before cooking them can remove some of the indigestible sugars in beans that produce gas during digestion.

Gas-forming foods also include cauliflower, broccoli, Brussels sprouts, cucumbers, red and green peppers, and onions. Fiber-rich foods can also be problematic in this regard. Gradually increasing the fiber content of your diet should keep this to a minimum, however.

Several digestive complaints can include flatulence as a symptom. For more information, refer to the sections in this book addressing food allergies, lactose intolerance, Crohn's disease, and irritable bowel syndrome.

Including active-culture yogurt in your diet can help normalize the bacterial residents in your intestinal tract and minimize gas. Taking supplements of the probiotic acidophilus achieves the same effect.

A class of herbs called carminatives work to quell excessive gas and ease painful spasms in the intestinal tract. Peppermint, fennel, and caraway are premier members of this class. Used alone or in combination, these herbs have been found in several studies to reduce gas and cramping.

Beneficial Roles of Intestinal Bacteria

The intestine is a very busy place. It's called home by more than 400 different species of bacteria. Fortunately, less than 1 percent of these bacteria are harmful. However, that 1 percent has the potential to cause anything from mild gastrointestinal upset to severe infection and even death. Consequently, your health depends on beneficial intestinal flora to keep the harmful bacteria at bay.

Individuals with flourishing colonies of good bacteria are better equipped to fight the excessive and dangerous growth of bad bacteria. This is because bacteria compete for "real estate" in the intestine for establishing colonies. When the intestine is full of large colonies of beneficial bacteria, a stray harmful germ cannot multiply because it can't find any unoccupied space on the intestinal wall.

Probiotics are "friendly bacteria," such as bifidobacteria and *Lactobacillus acidophilus,* that promote good health by limiting the growth of harmful bacteria, aiding good digestion, boosting immune function, and increasing resistance to infection. Fructooligosaccharides (FOS) are naturally occurring carbohydrates that cannot be digested or absorbed by humans, but are used as fuel for these beneficial bacteria. As such, some supplements of probiotics include this helpful ingredient.

Probiotics are found in fermented dairy foods and have been used as a folk remedy for hundreds, if not thousands, of years. Yogurt is the traditional source of beneficial bacteria; however, different brands of yogurt can vary greatly in their bacteria strain and potency. Many processed yogurts don't contain any active bacteria; check the label to see if "active cultures" are present. Dietary supplements supplying active and beneficial strains of bacteria are available.

When to Use Probiotics

There are numerous times that taking probiotics can be helpful. Topping the list is when diarrhea strikes. Diarrhea can have any number of causes, but it always has the same result on intestinal microorganisms—it flushes them out, leaving the body vulnerable to opportunistic infections. Replacing the flushed out healthy bacteria with probiotic supplements is important in preventing new infections. Probiotics can also help prevent the occurrence of diarrhea in the first place. A type of yeast called *Saccharomyces boulardii* has also been shown to prevent and treat diarrhea caused by some infectious organisms. When on vacation, supplementing with probiotics can greatly reduce the chances that you'll come down with a case of traveler's diarrhea. Another important time to take probiotics is during and after the use of antibiotic medications.

In addition, probiotics are a source of lactase enzyme, which is needed to digest milk, but lacking in lactose-intolerant individuals. Symptoms of irritable bowel syndrome may be alleviated by increased probiotic intake.

Colon Therapy

Cleansing the bowels has been relied upon as a primary healing tool for a myriad of diseases for thousands of years. It has gone in and out of favor over the years. In the early 1900s, there was a flurry of research showing it to be beneficial for many health problems, but the research field has really languished since then, in part because

pharmacology and medical technology moved
to the forefront in its place. Enemas and laxatives
can both be used to clean out the colon, although many practitioners rely on the less time-
consuming suggestion of laxatives as opposed
to irrigating with an enema.

Enemas can be used during times of constipation to remove feces. Other times that enemas
are appropriate are for cleansing the rectum in
preparation for an examination or surgical procedure or to administer therapeutic
substances. Habitual use of enemas
to resolve constipation can actually
make the problem even worse as the
body comes to rely on the enema.
Consequently, they should be used
only as a last resort for treatment
of constipation.

Enema
*The insertion
of a solution
into the rectum
and lower
intestine.*

Part of the reason that enemas have fallen out
of favor are legitimate concerns about maintaining a sterile procedure so that infection is not
introduced to the colon, potential damage to
delicate colon tissues, and electrolyte imbal-
ances. Enemas should not be administered to
anyone who recently had colon or rectal surgery,
a heart attack, or who suffers from an unknown
abdominal condition or an irregular heartbeat.

Enema or colon irrigation equipment should
be used according to the directions on the label.
Choose equipment with flexible tubes to reduce
the chances of damaging the rectum. In addition,
it is very important to disinfect the equipment
between uses.

There are high and low enemas, depending
on whether the goal is to cleanse as much of the
bowel as possible, or if only the lower bowel is
to be irrigated with fluid. Oil-retention enemas
lubricate the rectum and soften stool. A health
practitioner should be consulted if you are inter-

ested in learning the proper techniques for enemas or if you want to irrigate the colon with medications or herbs.

Bottom Line

- Fiber is essential in the prevention of diverticulitis. The herbs chamomile and peppermint can help heal an intestine that is bothered by diverticulitis.

- Fiber deserves another mention in the prevention of hemorrhoids. Witch hazel and vitamin C might help after the fact.

- Intestinal gas might be less of a problem for those eating more probiotics. Peppermint, fennel, and caraway can help with symptoms.

CONCLUSION

You should now have a good understanding of the ins and outs of digestion, as well as the importance of diet and lifestyle for a smooth running digestive process.

You no longer have to suffer needlessly or put yourself at the mercy of conventional medications with serious side effects if your digestive process has gone haywire. There is any number of natural ways to make friends again with digestion—by altering your diet, by making positive lifestyle choices, and/or by taking dietary supplements.

By reading this book, you've taken an important step toward enhancing your health and well-being. Now, the next step is to go with your gut to choose the best diet, lifestyle, and supplements or herb that will maximize your health and minimize your health complaints. Your health is in your hands.

NATURAL
DIGESTIVE AIDS

ALOE
CONDITION: Constipation
DOSAGE: 50–200 mg of aloe latex per day.
SPECIAL NOTE: Do not take for more than 10 days.

ARTICHOKE
CONDITION: Irritable bowel syndrome
DOSAGE: 320-mg capsules, 4–6 times per day.

BANANA POWDER
CONDITION: Ulcer
DOSAGE: 2 capsules 4 times per day for 8 weeks.

BERBERINE-CONTAINING HERBS (goldenseal, goldthread, barberry, Oregon grape)
CONDITION: Parasitic infection
DOSAGE: 500 mg of berberine per day.
SPECIAL NOTE: Gastrointestinal distress could occur at higher intakes.

BILBERRY
CONDITION: Diarrhea
DOSAGE: 300 mg of herbal extract per day.
SPECIAL NOTE: Do not use fresh berries, as they can worsen diarrhea.

BITTER HERBS (artichoke, bitter orange, blessed thistle, centaury, gentian, greater celandine)
CONDITION: Indigestion
DOSAGE: Add 2 ml of tincture to a 6-ounce glass of water and sip it before a meal until the drink is finished.
SPECIAL NOTE: Do not take if you have heartburn, ulcer, or gastritis.

BLACKBERRY LEAVES
CONDITION: Diarrhea
DOSAGE: Drink several cups of tea per day.

BREWER'S YEAST
CONDITION: Diarrhea
DOSAGE: 1–2 tablespoons of the powder per day.

CALCIUM
CONDITION: Digestive cancer-risk reduction
DOSAGE: 1,250–2,000 mg per day.

CARAWAY
CONDITION: Gas, indigestion, irritable bowel syndrome
DOSAGE: Gas/indigestion: 3–5 drops of essential oil or 3–5 ml of tincture, taken in water 2–3 times per day before meals.
DOSAGE: Irritable bowel syndrome: 50 mg of enteric-coated oil, taken 3 times per day.

CAROB
CONDITION: Diarrhea
DOSAGE: 20 grams per day.

CASCARA
CONDITION: Constipation
DOSAGE: 20–30 mg of cascarosides in capsule form per day.
SPECIAL NOTE: Do not use long term, as the colon may become weakened.

CHAMOMILE
CONDITION: Crohn's disease, diverticulitis, heartburn, irritable bowel syndrome, ulcers
DOSAGE: Drink 3–4 cups of tea per day between meals.

CHLOROPHYLL
CONDITION: Constipation
DOSAGE: 100 mg, 2–3 times per day.

DIGESTIVE ENZYMES (proteases, lipases, amylases)
CONDITION: Celiac disease, indigestion
DOSAGE: Follow label directions, or take 1.5 grams of 9X potency with each meal daily.

EVENING PRIMROSE OIL
CONDITION: Irritable bowel syndrome
DOSAGE: Capsules supplying 400 mg of GLA per day.

FENNEL
CONDITION: Gas
DOSAGE: 3–5 drops of essential oil or 3–5 ml of tincture, taken in water 2–3 times per day before meals.

FENUGREEK

CONDITION: Constipation, diarrhea

DOSAGE: 2 teaspoons of the seeds per day.

SPECIAL NOTE: Take with plenty of water. Do not take more or abdominal distress could result.

FISH OIL

CONDITION: Crohn's disease, digestive cancer-risk reduction

DOSAGE: Crohn's disease: 2.7 grams of enteric-coated "free fatty acid" form of EPA/DHA per day.

DOSAGE: Cancer: Consume several servings of fish per week or take 2–3 grams of fish oil supplements per day.

SPECIAL NOTE: Take 100–400 IU of vitamin E to protect the oil from free-radical damage; some people experience upset stomach or "fishy" burps.

FLAXSEED

CONDITION: Constipation

DOSAGE: 1–3 tablespoons of whole or crushed flaxseed 2–3 times a day.

SPECIAL NOTE: Take with plenty of water.

FOLIC ACID

CONDITION: Crohn's disease, digestive cancer-risk reduction

DOSAGE: 400–800 mcg per day.

GAMMA-ORYZANOL

CONDITION: Gastritis

DOSAGE: 300 mg per day.

GARLIC

CONDITION: Digestive cancer-risk reduction, parasites, ulcer

DOSAGE: Add fresh garlic to cooking as desired, or take 600–900 mg of standardized garlic per day.

SPECIAL NOTE: Can cause heartburn and gas in some people.

GINGER

CONDITION: Indigestion, morning sickness, motion sickness, nausea/ vomiting

DOSAGE: 500 mg every 2–4 hours, as needed.

SPECIAL NOTE: Do not take if you have a history of gallstones.

GLUCOMANNAN

CONDITION: Constipation

DOSAGE: 3–4 grams per day.

SPECIAL NOTE: Take with plenty of water. Some people might experience more flatulence as the body adjusts to a higher fiber intake.

GLUTAMINE

CONDITION: Leaky gut syndrome, ulcer

DOSAGE: Leaky gut syndrome: 500–1,000 mg per day.

DOSAGE: Ulcer: 1,000 mg per day during the acute phase.

GREEN TEA (and black tea)

CONDITION: Crohn's disease, diarrhea, digestive cancer-risk reduction, food poisoning

DOSAGE: Drink several cups of caffeinated or decaf tea daily, as desired.

LACTASE

CONDITION: Lactose intolerance

DOSAGE: Take drops, tablets, or capsules, as directed on label.

LICORICE (DGL form)

CONDITION: Crohn's disease, indigestion, ulcers

DOSAGE: 1–2 chewable DGL tablets (250–500 mg per tablet) 15 minutes before meals and 1–2 hours before bedtime daily.

SPECIAL NOTE: Use the DGL form of licorice to prevent blood pressure from rising as with the non-DGL form.

MARSHMALLOW

CONDITION: Crohn's disease, diarrhea, ulcers

DOSAGE: 5–6 grams of herbal extract per day.

MILK THISTLE

CONDITION: Gallstones, liver health

DOSAGE: 420 mg of silymarin (the active constituent of milk thistle) per day.

SPECIAL NOTE: Can have a laxative effect.

PEPPERMINT

CONDITION: Crohn's disease, diverticulitis, gas, indigestion, irritable bowel syndrome

DOSAGE: Crohn's disease, diverticulitis, gas, and indigestion: Drink as a tea, as desired, or take 3–5 drops of essential oil or 3–5 ml of tincture, in water 2–3 times per day before meals.

DOSAGE: Irritable bowel syndrome: 90-mg enteric-coated oil, taken 3 times per day.

SPECIAL NOTE: Peppermint oil can cause burning and GI upset in some people.

PHOSPHATIDYLCHOLINE

CONDITION: Gallstones, liver health

DOSAGE: 300–2,000 mg per day.

PROBIOTICS

CONDITION: Crohn's disease, diarrhea, digestive cancer-risk reduction, food poisoning, gas

DOSAGE: Eat active culture yogurt or supplement with 1–2 billion colony forming units (CFUs) per day of probiotic bacteria; 8 grams per day of FOS.

PSYLLIUM

CONDITION: Constipation, diarrhea

DOSAGE: Constipation: 7.5 grams of psyllium seeds or 5 grams of psyllium husks, 1–2 times per day

DOSAGE: Diarrhea: 5 grams of psyllium husks 3 times per day or up to 30 grams of the whole seeds per day.

SPECIAL NOTE: Take with plenty of water. Do not use if you have asthma.

PUMPKIN SEEDS

CONDITION: Parasites

DOSAGE: 200–400 grams per day.

RED RASPBERRY LEAVES

CONDITION: Diarrhea

DOSAGE: Drink several cups of tea per day.

SACCHAROMYCES BOULARDII

CONDITION: Diarrhea

DOSAGE: 500 mg 4 times per day.

SELENIUM

CONDITION: Digestive cancer-risk reduction

DOSAGE: 100–200 mcg per day.

SENNA

CONDITION: Constipation

DOSAGE: Follow label directions, generally 20–60 mg of sennosides per day.

SPECIAL NOTE: Do not use for more than 10 days or dependency can develop.

SLIPPERY ELM

CONDITION: Crohn's disease, diarrhea, indigestion

DOSAGE: 500-mg capsules, 3–4 times per day.

VITAMIN A

CONDITION: Digestive cancer-risk reduction, ulcer

DOSAGE: 5,000–10,000 IU per day.

SPECIAL NOTE: Pregnant women should limit intake to 7,500 IU per day.

VITAMIN B$_6$

CONDITION: Morning sickness

DOSAGE: 30 mg per day.

SPECIAL NOTE: Do not take more than 200 mg per day.

VITAMIN B$_{12}$

CONDITION: Crohn's disease

DOSAGE: 2 mcg per day.

VITAMIN C

CONDITION: Digestive cancer-risk reduction, gallstones, hemorrhoids, liver health

DOSAGE: 500–1,500 mg per day.

SPECIAL NOTE: Nausea, diarrhea, and stomach cramping can occur in some individuals; if so, reduce dosage.

VITAMIN E

CONDITION: Digestive cancer-risk reduction

DOSAGE: 100–400 IU per day.

ZINC

CONDITION: Crohn's disease, leaky gut syndrome, ulcer

DOSAGE: 25–50 mg per day.

SPECIAL NOTE: Do not take more than 150 mg per day.

APPENDIX B

GUIDED TOUR OF THE DIGESTIVE SYSTEM

Here's a refresher about the basic process of digestion. The digestive system has several parts that all work in concert for the goal of digesting and absorbing food. The breakdown of food occurs in the stomach (gastro) and the intestine, which is why it is also called the gastrointestinal (GI) tract. The GI tract can be thought of as an approximately 16.5 feet long tube extending from the mouth to the anus. It includes the mouth, esophagus, stomach, small intestine, pancreas, gallbladder, liver, and large intestine.

The whole system starts to work as soon as a bite of food enters the mouth. The process of chewing mashes the food into smaller, more manageable pieces. Next, the food is swallowed, meaning that it travels down the esophagus—a tube that connects the mouth to the stomach. A series of wavelike contractions keep the food moving down to the stomach and through the rest of the GI tract.

Once in the stomach, the powerful muscles of the stomach churn the food, breaking it into smaller and smaller pieces. Gastric juices produced by the glands lining the stomach mix with the food particles. These juices contain pepsin, an enzyme that begins to digest proteins, and hydrochloric acid to acidify the stomach. Very few foods are actually absorbed in the stomach— only alcohol, simple sugars, and some medications—the rest of the nutrient absorption takes place later in the digestive tract.

The next stop is the small intestine, where the majority of food absorption takes place. Digestive enzymes from the pancreas and intestinal lining, as well as bile from the gallbladder and liver, continue to prepare the food for absorption. Billions of specialized cells line the small intestine and absorb the end-products of digestion: amino acids from protein, sugar from carbohydrates, fatty acids from fats, cholesterol, vitamins, and minerals. What's left over—water, undigested fibers, some minerals, bile, and waste products—is shuttled to the large intestine. Most of the water is reabsorbed, and the rest of the large intestine's contents are excreted from the body as stool.

The above description of digestion is what happens in an ideal world. In the real world, there are many pitfalls and problems that result in poor nutrient absorption, constipation, diarrhea, bloating, gas, and a host of other digestive problems.

SELECTED REFERENCES

Bertram B, Bartsch H. Cancer prevention with green tea: reality and wishful thinking. *Wien Med Wochenschr* 2002;152(5-6):153–8.

Duffield-Lillico AJ, Reid ME, Turnbull BW, et al. Baseline characteristics and the effect of selenium supplementation on cancer incidence in a randomized clinical trial: a summary report of the nutritional prevention of cancer trial. *Cancer Epidemiol Biomarkers Prev* 2002;11(7):630–9.

Fernandez E, Chatenound L, La Vecchia C, et al. Fish consumption and cancer risk. *Am J Clin Nutr* 1999; 70:85–90.

Freise J, Kohler S. Peppermint oil-caraway oil fixed combination in non-ulcer dyspepsia—comparison of the effects of enteric preparations. *Pharmazie* 1999;54:210–15.

Gao C, Takezaki T, Ding J, et al. Protective effect of allium vegetables against both esophageal and stomach cancer: a simultaneous case-referent study of a high-epidemic area in Jiangsu Province, China. *Jpn J Cancer Res* 1999;90:614–21.

Gullo L. Indication for pancreatic enzyme treatment in non-pancreatic digestive diseases. *Digestion* 1993;54 (suppl 2):43–7.

Gupta P, Andrew H, Kirschner BS, et al. Is *lactobacillus GG* helpful in children with Crohn's disease? Results of a preliminary, open-label study. *J Pediatr Gastroenterol Nutr* 2000;31:453–7.

Guslandi M, Mezzi G, Sorghi M, et al. *Saccharomyces boulardii* in maintenance treatment of Crohn's disease. *Dig Dis Sci* 2000;45:1462–4.

Kaneda Y, Torii M, Tanaka T, Aikawa M. In vitro effects of berberine sulphate on the growth and structure of

Entamoeba histolytica, Giardia lamblia and *Tricho-monas vaginalis. Ann Trop Med Parasitol* 1991;85: 417–25.

Kraft K. Artichoke leaf extract—recent findings reflecting effects on lipid metabolism, liver and gastrointestinal tracts. *Phytomedicine* 1997;4:370–8 [review].

Laugier R, et al. Changes in pancreatic exocrine secretion with age: Pancreatic exocrine secretion does decrease in the elderly. *Digestion* 1991;50:202–11.

Meydani M, Meydani M. Nutrition interventions in aging and age-associated disease. *Proc Nutr Soc* 2002;61(2):165–71.

Passmore AP, Wilson-Davies K, Flanagan PG, et al. Chronic constipation in long stay elderly patients: a comparison of lactulose and senna-fiber combination. *BMJ* 1993;307:769–71.

Patriarca G, Schiavino D, Nucera E, et al. Food allergy in children: results of a standardized protocol for oral desensitization. *Hepatogastroenterology* 1998;45:52–8.

Ribenfeld D, Borzone L. Randomized double-blind study comparing ginger (Zintona(r)) with dimenhydrinate in motion sickness. *Healthnotes Rev Complementary Integrative Med* 1999;6:98–101.

Ritter R, Schatton WFH, et al. Clinical trial on standardized celandine extract in patients with functional epigastric complaints: Results of placebo-controlled double-blind trial. *Comp Ther Med* 1993;1:189–93.

Scarpignato C, Rampal P. Prevention and treatment of traveler's diarrhea: A clinical pharmacological approach. *Chemotherapy* 1995;41:48–81.

Srinivassan U, Leonard N, Jones E, et al. Absence of oats toxicity in adult coeliac disease. *BMJ* 1996; 313:1300–1.

Staianno A, Simeone D, Giudice ED, et al. Effect of the dietary fiber glucomannan on chronic constipation in neurologically impaired children. *J Pediatr* 2000;136: 41–5.

Sturniolo GC, Di Leo V, Fettonato A, et al. Zinc supplementation tightens "leaky gut" in Crohn's disease. *Inflamm Bowel Dis* 2001;7:94–8.

Suarez F, Levitt MD, Adshead J, Barkin JS. Pancreatic supplements reduce symptomatic response of healthy subjects to a high fat meal. *Dig Dis Sci* 1999;44: 1317–21.

Walker AF, Middleton RW, Petrowicz O. Artichoke leaf extract reduces symptoms of irritable bowel syndrome in a post-marketing surveillance study. *Phytother Res* 2001;15:58–61.

Wright CW, Phillipson JD. Natural products and the development of selective antiprotozoal drugs. *Phytother Res* 1990;4:127–39 [review].

OTHER
RESOURCES

GreatLife Magazine
Consumer magazine with articles on vitamins, minerals, herbs, and foods.
Available for free at many health and natural food stores.

Let's Live Magazine
Consumer magazine with emphasis on the health benefits of vitamins, minerals, and herbs.

Customer service:
1-800-676-4333
P.O. Box 74908
Los Angeles, CA 90004
Subscriptions: 12 issues per year, $19.95 in the U.S.; $31.95 outside the U.S.

Physical Magazine
Magazine oriented to body builders and other serious athletes.

Customer service:
1-800-676-4333
P.O. Box 74908
Los Angeles, CA 90004
Subscriptions: 12 issues per year, $19.95 in the U.S.; $31.95 outside the U.S.

The Nutrition Reporter™ newsletter
Monthly newsletter that summarizes recent medical research on vitamins, minerals, and herbs.

Customer service:
P.O. Box 30246
Tucson, AZ 85751-0246
e-mail: jack@thenutritionreporter.com
www.nutritionreporter.com
Subscriptions: $26 per year (12 issues) in the U.S.;
$32 U.S. or $48 CNC for Canada; $38 for other
countries.

National Cancer Institute
www.nci.nih.gov

The American Gastroenterological Association
7910 Woodmont Avenue, 7th Floor
Bethesda, MD 20814
301-654-2055

The American College of Gastroenterology
P.O. Box 3099
Alexandria, VA 22302
(703) 820-7400

National Digestive Diseases Information
Clearinghouse
2 Information Way
Bethesda, MD 20892-3570
E-mail: nddic@info.niddk.nih.gov

INDEX